Women and schizophrenia

This comprehensive review of a complex area is as much about women as it is about schizophrenia, encompassing the biological, endocrinological, epidemiological, reproductive, psychological and social aspects of schizophrenia as experienced by women. Femaleness impacts significantly on the onset and nature of schizophrenia suffered by women: the female brain develops more rapidly than the male; estrogens produce antipsychotic effects; the female brain ages differently from the male, with a massive preponderance of female very-late-onset schizophrenia which may be related to a relative excess of dopamine D_2 receptors.

An international multidisciplinary team of clinicians and mental health researchers review past and current literature, assess the sex-specific issues and evaluate their therapeutic, clinical and social implications for more appropriate and effective treatments of schizophrenia in women now and in the future. This book is essential reading for all clinicians, practitioners and researchers involved with mental health and also with women's health.

Professor David Castle is the Clinical Director of Mental Health Services at Fremantle Hospital in Australia. He is the author of over 100 papers dealing in the main with the impact of sex on schizophrenia and late-onset schizophrenia.

Professor John McGrath is Director of the Queensland Centre for Schizophrenia Research, a multidisciplinary group focusing on the causes of schizophrenia.

Professor Jayashri Kulkarni is Director of the Monash University Research Centre for Women's Mental Health where she is involved in several clinical research projects looking at treatments, outcomes and quality of life, including one study examining the use of estrogen as a treatment for schizophrenia.

Women and schizophrenia

Edited by

David J. Castle

John McGrath

and

Jayashri Kulkarni

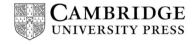

CAMBRIDGE
UNIVERSITY PRESS

PUBLISHED BY THE PRESS SYNDICATE OF THE UNIVERSITY OF CAMBRIDGE
The Pitt Building, Trumpington Street, Cambridge, United Kingdom

CAMBRIDGE UNIVERSITY PRESS
The Edinburgh Building, Cambridge CB2 2RU, UK   http://www.cup.cam.ac.uk
40 West 20th Street, New York, NY 10011–4211, USA   http://www.cup.org
10 Stamford Road, Oakleigh, Melbourne 3166, Australia
Ruiz de Alarcón 13, 28014 Madrid, Spain

First published 2000
Reprinted 2000

Printed in the United Kingdom at the University Press, Cambridge

Typeset in Minion 11/14.5 pt [v n]

A catalogue record for this book is available from the British Library

Library of Congress Cataloguing in Publication data

Women and schizophrenia / edited by David J. Castle, John McGrath, Jayashri Kulkarni.
    p.   cm.
Includes index.
ISBN 0 521 78617 7 (pb)
1. Schizophrenia.   2. Women – Diseases.   3. Women – Mental health.   I. Castle, David J.
II. McGrath, John, 1958–   III. Kulkarni, Jayashri, 1958–
[DNLM: 1. Schizophrenia. 2. Women. WM203 W872 2000]
RC514.W613 2000
616.89'82'0082–dc21   99-057083

ISBN 0 521 78617 7 paperback

Contents

Contributors

Joanne Barkla
Research Psychiatrist
Queensland Centre for Schizophrenia Research
Wolston Park Hospital
Wacol, Q4076
Australia

David J. Castle
Clinical Associate Professor
Clinical Director
Mental Health Services
Fremantle Hospital & Health Service
PO Box 480
Fremantle, WA 6959
Australia

George Fink
MRC Brain Metabolism Unit
Department of Pharmacology
University of Edinburgh
1 George Square
Edinburgh, EH8 9JZ
Scotland

Paul Fitzgerald
Consultant Psychiatrist
Department of Psychiatry
Dandenong Psychiatric Hospital
134 Cleeland Street
Dandenong, VIC 3175
Australia

Jill M. Goldstein
Harvard Institute of Psychiatric Epidemiology and
Genetics
74 Fenwood Road
Boston, MA 02115
USA

Jenny Hearle
Research Associate
Queensland Centre for Schizophrenia Research
Wacol, Q4076
Australia

Jayashri Kulkarni
Associate Professor
Department of Psychiatry
Dandenong Psychiatric Hospital
134 Cleeland Street
Dandenong, VIC 3175
Australia

Richard R.J. Lewine
Department of Psychiatry and Behavioral Sciences
Emory School of Medicine
1701 Uppergate Drive, NE
Atlanta, GA 30322
USA

John McGrath
Associate Professor
Director
Queensland Centre for Schizophrenia Research
Wolston Park Hospital
Wacol, Q4076
Australia

Robin MacGregor Murray
Professor
Kings College Hospital
Institute of Psychiatry
De Crespigny Park
London, SE5 8AF
UK

Mary V. Seeman
Professor
Tapscott Chair in Schizophrenia Studies
University of Toronto
Centre for Addiction and Mental Health
Clarke Division
250 College Street
Toronto, Ontario, M5T 1R8, Canada

Foreword

I am delighted to recommend this highly readable book. Firstly, it is an extremely important subject. Secondly, I learnt a lot from the nine chapters, and I have no doubt that others will do the same. Thirdly, and more parochially, two of the editors (D.C. and J.McG.) are former members of my own department whose subsequent work on schizophrenia I have followed with great interest.

Why write (or read) a book on schizophrenia in women when there are no similar books on schizophrenia in men? The answer is that the prototypical patient with a diagnosis of schizophrenia is male, and most studies of people with schizophrenia have contained many more men than women. Indeed, there has been a recent trend in some fields, such as functional neuroimaging, to study only males (in an effort to reduce heterogeneity). The result is that many discussions and recommendations about schizophrenia are in fact about schizophrenia in males.

Of course, there remains considerable controversy about the very existence of schizophrenia as a distinct entity. Even Kraepelin, who invented the concept (initially termed dementia praecox), later expressed the view that schizophrenia was merely a provisional category, and that the dichotomous classification of psychosis might some day be replaced by a better system. Unfortunately, we have not yet reached that point. In the meantime, therefore, in the search for more knowledge, there is a lot to be said for investigating those facts about schizophrenia which appear to be most consistent across cultures; and among these, differences between male and female sufferers are pre-eminent.

Dr Castle and his colleagues throw a penetrating light on the data showing that females with a diagnosis of schizophrenia have, on average, better childhood function, a later onset of illness, and a better response to treatment than their male counterparts. Why? Are the schizophrenia-like disorders that afflict men and women essentially different? Do, for example, many females who receive a diagnosis of schizophrenia really suffer from an illness which is driven by mood disturbance and in which the schizophrenic symptoms are secondary phenomena? Alternatively, is it that women in general, and not just women diagnosed as having schizophrenia, tend to have fewer negative behaviours, more comprehensible speech, and more social skill than their male counterparts? Readers will not be presented with a definitive answer but they will see a clear presentation of the different points of view, and can make up their own minds.

The editors also introduce a number of relatively new topics. These include the question of whether hormone replacement therapy has a place in the treatment of women with onset of schizophrenia later in life. Secondly, the important public health issue of ensuring that women with schizophrenia have the best possible antenatal and perinatal care lest the increased genetic risk of their offspring is compounded by cerebral insult. Finally, the increasingly common question of how best to help mothers with schizophrenia to provide an optimum upbringing for their children.

I wish I had thought of the idea of a book on this important but neglected topic. Sadly, I didn't, but reading this one is the next best thing!

Robin MacGregor Murray
Professor of Psychiatry
Institute of Psychiatry
London

Preface

This book is as much about women as it is about schizophrenia. It takes as its premise the notion that understanding differences between women and men in terms of biological, psychological and social domains can inform our understanding of gender differences in schizophrenia, but more broadly schizophrenia as a disorder. Specifically, those particular vulnerabilities and strengths which women show, relative to men, are explored and brought to bear on an exploration of gender differences in schizophrenia.

For example, the fact that the female brain develops more rapidly than that of the male, leaving it less vulnerable to early developmental insult, could explain the relative protection of females from the severe early dementia praecox type of schizophrenia, postulated to be consequent upon neurodevelopmental damage. On the other hand, the antidopaminergic properties of estrogens are explored in some detail, and the animal and clinical experiments showing this to translate into antipsychotic effects are reviewed. This lays the ground for consideration of a possible protective effect of female sex hormones against the onset of schizophrenia in premenopausal women. The price is paid once estrogen levels fall at the menopause, and a second peak of onset of schizophrenia is seen in females at this age. This has important potential therapeutic implications.

Further, the fact that female brains age differently from those of males is important in explaining the massive female preponderance in a very-late schizophrenia (late paraphrenia, usually with an onset after the age of 60). Differential rates of loss of dopamine D_2 receptors between the sexes, with females beginning life with a relative deficit, but having a relative excess in later life, are of particular importance here, and might also account for the particular vulnerability of elderly women to tardive dyskinesia upon exposure to neuroleptic medication.

The book also serves to outline the psychosocial context of women with schizophrenia. Inevitably the views presented here are largely reflective of the situation in so-called developed or industrialized countries, but issues such as marriage (or its equivalent) and childbirth are part of all human societies. Increasingly it is important for the male-dominated medical profession to be aware of women's issues in these domains, as the recognition thereof will allow more appropriate, accessible, acceptable and ultimately effective interventions to be brought to bear to help women with schizophrenia. We trust this book will assist in this process.

David J. Castle

August 1999

Introduction and overview

John McGrath, David J. Castle and Jayashri Kulkarni

Weighing up the differences and commonalities between women with schizophrenia and men with schizophrenia, it would be fair to say that men and women with schizophrenia have more in common than they have points of distinction. Why then, edit a book about women with schizophrenia?

- Epidemiology, genetics and neuroscience highlight differences between men and women with schizophrenia that may illuminate causal mechanisms.
- Biological factors associated with being a woman can modify clinical outcomes in schizophrenia. This type of research may provide direction for developing improved treatments for the disorder.
- Clinicians need to be mindful that factors related to gender may have an impact on treatment choices.
- The impact of schizophrenia on women and their role in society warrant special attention. Gender modifies the impairment and disablement associated with schizophrenia. In turn, the interaction between this disablement and sociocultural factors results in particular handicaps for women with schizophrenia.

The aim of this book is to examine selected issues related to the interactions between schizophrenia and being female. One could equally write a book about the special issues for men with schizophrenia; however, the focus on women allows us to redress the relative lack of attention to the special needs of women. This book will be of interest to clinicians involved in the care of women with schizophrenia, students from the mental health professions, researchers and service planners.

Overview of chapters

Chapter 2 reviews issues related to the development, organization and degeneration of the human female brain which are relevant to schizophrenia. Much evidence has accumulated in the last two decades that suggests that subtle deviations in brain development may be associated with adult-onset psychoses. Sex hormones play an important role in the development of the brain, and expressly influence the definition of gender-specificity. Particular developmental and organizational parameters of the female brain might influence both susceptibility to, and expression of, schizophrenia. Similarly, the degenerative trajectory of the female brain differs from that of the male, and might explain the female preponderance in late-onset schizophrenia.

This chapter also provides an overview of differences between girls and boys in performance on certain neuropsychological tasks and outlines their differential susceptibility to, and expression of, mental disorders in childhood and adolescence. This allows the further consideration of gender differences in schizophrenia to be placed in the wider developmental context.

Epidemiology can inform much of the debate regarding gender differences in schizophrenia and related disorders, and Chapter 3 summarizes selected aspects of the epidemiology of schizophrenia that are salient to women. One of the most consistent findings in schizophrenia research relates to the differences in age of onset between men and women. Furthermore, it is increasingly clear that age-at-onset curves for males and females are not isomorphic. Any coherent theory of schizophrenia must explain these findings.

Some of these key factors are returned to in Chapter 4, which expands the discussion by examining clinical aspects of schizophrenia in women. These include better premorbid functioning, more affective and less negative symptomatology and a more benign longitudinal course compared with males with schizophrenia. These issues again need to be incorporated into any explanatory model of gender differences in schizophrenia.

Chapter 5 provides a special focus on hormones and psychosis. This is an area with a long research history, but is one where only recently have methodologically sound studies been performed. Of particular interest are reports of an association between estrogen levels and psychosis and the potential therapeutic benefit of estrogens in schizophrenia. Clinical guidelines for the use of adjunctive estrogens in this context are also provided.

Chapter 6 examines selected issues related to reproduction and antenatal care in women with schizophrenia. Opportunities exist to improve antenatal service to women with schizophrenia that could result in improved clinical outcomes for the mother and offspring. However, service providers need to follow through with services to assist mothers with schizophrenia. Some of the special issues related to motherhood are addressed in Chapter 7.

One of the motives for editing this book is the belief that a more explicit understanding of women's issues in schizophrenia can usefully inform treatment. Chapter 8 takes a broad approach to treatment issues for females with schizophrenia, encompassing biological, psychological and social domains. The chapter thus reflects upon, and provides a practical therapeutic response to, many of the issues raised elsewhere in the book.

The final chapter provides a summary of the defining features that have emerged with respect to women and schizophrenia, highlighting what is now at the 'cutting edge' of work in this area; these include brain imaging and molecular genetic research. This context provides an opportunity to delineate directions for future research into the causes of, and therapeutic implications for, gender differences in schizophrenia.

Caveats

The chapters in this book are focused on women who have schizophrenia, but there are other related issues that link schizophrenia and women. For example, mothers of people with schizophrenia were cast as 'schizophrenogenic' by past research. While these theories are now discredited, there is evidence to show that obstetric complications in the mother can increase the risk of schizophrenia in the offspring. It is important that such knowledge results in better obstetric care for women with schizophrenia, rather than having as a consequence further pejorative labelling.

Another area that warrants mention is the role women play as informal carers for people with schizophrenia. This field of research has been neglected, but clinical experience in many societies suggest that mothers, wives and daughters bear the brunt of providing disability support for their relative with schizophrenia. Mental health professionals need to acknowledge and validate the important roles women play in the care of those with schizophrenia. Service planners should examine ways to deliver support to assist women in these roles.

Women also provide professional care to individuals with schizophrenia, and many schizophrenia researchers are women. It seems that in many countries there are gender imbalances that shift across the spectrum of health care (e.g. nurses, doctors, case managers, team leaders, academics, bureaucrats). We need to remain mindful that these imbalances may subtly distort clinical and research perspectives.

We urge the reader to exercise caution in the application of any treatment recommendations contained in this book. It is becoming increasingly apparent that clinicians need an evidence base that can rapidly incorporate new knowledge – textbooks can provide the best available evidence at the time of writing, but it is probable that some of the treatment recommendations will very quickly be out of date.

In conclusion, we hope that this book provides information that can translate into both immediate and longer-term gains for women with schizophrenia. It is clear that there are gaps in current services that can be addressed in the short term. We also hope that gender issues can act as a prism through which we can refract the 'light' of schizophrenia into its component parts, and that researchers can eventually use this knowledge to reduce the incidence of, and disability associated with, this group of disorders.

2

Sex differences in brain development, organization, and degeneration: are they relevant to sex differences in schizophrenia?

David J. Castle

This chapter reviews gender differences in the development, organization and degeneration of the human brain, looking also at the behavioural consequences of such gender differences, and attempting to tease apart biological from psychosocial determinants of male and female behaviour and neuropsychological performance. Of course, there is no strict dichotomy between biological and psychosocial determinants of behaviour, and gender differences in human behaviour and functioning are neither exclusively biologically, nor exclusively socially, determined. What is clear, however, is that throughout the animal kingdom, certain behaviours, expressly those related to reproduction, are sexually dimorphic (see Pilgrim & Reisert, 1992). Furthermore, certain brain structures are sexually dimorphic, and there are gender differences in performance on some neuropsychological tasks. And from a longitudinal perspective, the brains of males and females differ from each other in subtle but important ways, in terms of both development and degeneration. Such parameters need to be considered in any analysis of gender differences in schizophrenia.

We begin this chapter with an overview of sexual dimorphism of the human brain, and move on to a consideration of gender differences in brain development. We then review gender differences in neuropsychological functioning and cerebral laterality, progressing to a consideration of behavioural differences between boys and girls, placing these in a developmental framework. Finally, we provide an overview of gender differences in brain degenerative processes.

Sexual dimorphism in brain structures

Sexual dimorphisms in brain structures have been most dramatically demonstrated in animals. For example, in the male songbird the size of the region of the brain involved in production of song (a primarily male behaviour) is five to six times larger than in females (Nottenbohm & Arnold, 1976). In rats, the preoptic area of the hypothalamus is much larger in the male, so much so that the area has been called the 'sexually dimorphic preoptic area' (Gorski et al., 1980). It has been shown that this size discrepancy is largely consequent upon testosterone exposure during the so-called critical period of brain development (see later); exposure later in development results in a female-like nucleus. Subsequent reports have shown sexual dimorphism of this brain area in other animals, including guinea-pigs, gerbils and ferrets.

In humans, too, there is sexual dimorphism of the preoptic area. Thus, Swaab & Fliers (1985) described larger size of the nucleus in males; there were also differences in cell count, and histological appearance, between male and female brains. Of interest, though, is that the discrepancy in cell numbers between men and women varies with age, such that before the age of 10 the nucleus is sexually monomorphic; the dimorphism peaks in young adulthood; and cell numbers decline rapidly after the age of 50 in men and 70 in women. The precise basis for these developmental and degenerative differences between the sexes is not clear (Breedlove, 1994).

Other sexual dimorphisms in the human brain have been less consistently reported, and the interpretation of such differences that have been found has been difficult. For example, the male human brain is both larger and heavier than that of females; the difference is present at birth, although it becomes more pronounced in adulthood. However, most of this discrepancy can be accounted for by differences in body size and surface area.

Investigating gender differences in cortical structures, Haug (1984) found a higher density of neurones in the orbital area of females than in males. Also, the planum temporale shows right–left asymmetry in shape much more commonly in males than in females (Wada et al., 1975). The latter finding is of particular interest in terms of psychosis, in that it has been proposed (Crow, 1994) that schizophrenia is consequent upon abnormal cerebral lateralization (see later) and there have been reports of planum temporale asymmetry in patients with schizophrenia. In terms of gender, Reite et al. (1997) performed magnetic source imaging in 20 schizophrenia patients (nine female) and 20 controls. The male patient group showed less asymmetry of the 100 ms latency auditory evoked field component (M-100) than controls, whilst the females showed more significant asymmetry.

Also of potential relevance to schizophrenia are reports of gender differences in certain subcortical structures (notably the hippocampus), which have attracted considerable interest in attempts to understand the neuroanatomical basis for schizophrenic symptomatology. Thus, at least in voles, the hippocampus is consistently larger in males, while in rats the hippocampal–dentate complex shows sex differential laterality effects (Diamond, 1989).

There is also some evidence – albeit conflicting – of corpus callosum differences between the sexes; this is discussed in more detail below. Gender differences in certain limbic structures have also been reported, but tend to be subtle and somewhat inconsistent.

Brain development and the impact of testosterone

The basis of sexual differentiation appears largely to be determined by the presence or absence of the Y chromosome and, more particularly, of the hormone testosterone. Thus, in the presence of testosterone the brain develops certain 'male' characteristics, whilst the absence of this hormone allows the brain to continue to develop in a 'female' way.

In the male fetus, the developing testes start to secrete testosterone at intrauterine day 18 in the rat, coinciding with week 9 in humans. The timing of this testosterone surge has been equated with a proposed critical period for the influence of testosterone on the developing brain, encompassing weeks 9–18 of intrauterine development in humans (Finegan et al., 1988). Testosterone is actually aromatized to estrogen once it enters the brain so that, paradoxically, the characteristic 'male' brain owes its sexual dimorphism to a 'female' hormone. There appear to be two main mechanisms whereby testosterone and estrogen exert their effects on the brain, namely by influencing axonal growth and synaptogenesis, and by programmed cell death; these processes result in permanent changes in neuronal circuitry and organization (Pilgrim & Reisert, 1992). In this scenario, the female brain has been seen as the 'default pathway' in that its development follows that which would occur in the absence of testosterone.

The impact of testosterone exposure on the developing brain can be determined, in part at least, by experiments where either genetic males lack testosterone or genetic females are exposed to testosterone during the critical period. In rats, castration experiments have shown that male reproductive behaviour can be made 'female-like', and that normal gender-specific morphological differences in hypothalamic and limbic structures can be attenuated. Conversely, female guinea-pigs exposed to testosterone during the critical period show a lack of normal female sexual behaviour (Phoenix et al., 1959).

In humans, reliance has been placed on 'natural experiments' to determine these influences. Thus, females with congenital adrenal hyperplasia, where a defect in adrenal enzymes results in plasma androgen levels intermediate between normal males and females, are more likely as children to be tomboys, and to prefer toys usually favoured by boys (Berenbaum & Hines, 1992). There are also reports of more male-like neuropsychological performance in such individuals (Resnick et al., 1986). Similarly, women exposed *in utero* to the estrogenic compound diethylstilbestrol tend to show more lateralized functioning on a dichotic listening task than their unexposed sisters, indicating a masculinizing effect of the aromatized metabolites of androgen (Hines, 1982; Breedlove, 1994).

Conversely, men with idiopathic hypogonadotrophic hypogonadism have been shown to perform less well than normal controls or than men with acquired hypogonadism (i.e. where *in utero* testosterone exposure would have been at normal male levels) on tests of spatial ability (usually a particular strength for males, as discussed below). In these individuals there appears to be a negative correlation between testicular volume and spatial ability performance (Hier & Crowley, 1982).

It is as well to point out, however, that factors beside testosterone appear to be required for the full realization of 'maleness' in the human brain. Thus, Reisert & Pilgrim (1991) showed that sex-specific neural cultures of catecholaminergic neurones exhibit sex-specific morphological and functional sex differences even in the absence of testosterone. These authors concluded that there must be some inherent sex-specific genetic programming taking place, and that 'a cascade of cell-intrinsic and cell-extrinsic events is needed to establish a fully developed male or female brain'.

Some of the cell-intrinsic differences are presumably genetically mediated. Indeed, several genes for brain growth and development must be located on the sex chromosomes, as evidenced by the large number of known X linked mental retardation syndromes (Schwartz, 1993). Females have two X chromosomes, and males one, whilst males have male-specific genes on the Y chromosome. In order to have a differential effect, some X linked genes must escape the normal inactivation of most genes on the second X chromosome in females (a process called dosage compensation); thus, in the absence of dosage compensation there would be a greater amount of gene product in females than males. Y-linked genes might also influence brain development and organization.

Gender differences in neuropsychological functioning, cerebral laterality and language

It has long been held that men and women differ in terms of neuropsychological functioning. Eysenck (quoted by Ames, 1991) stated that:

men exceed women in visuospatial ability, of perceiving patterns as a whole and, consequently, at such practical skills as map reading and mechanics. Girls learn to talk earlier than boys do and articulate better and possess a more extensive vocabulary at all ages. They write and spell better, their grammar is better and they construct sentences better.

Kimura (1992) has reviewed gender differences in neuropsychological functioning. She concluded that males, on average, perform better than females on tests requiring imaginal rotation or other manipulation of objects; on tests of mathematical reasoning; on navigating through a route; and on target-directed motor skills. Females, on the other hand, tend to outperform males on tests of perceptual speed; arithmetic calculation; recalling landmarks from a route; and at certain precision manual tasks. Furthermore, girls tend to excel in tests of verbal fluency, in comparison with boys of the same age (McGee, 1982).

In broad terms, in humans, the right cerebral hemisphere is concerned with visuospatial skills, and verbal ability is mediated by the left hemisphere.

More specifically, the left hemisphere is thought to excel in areas of intellectual, rational, verbal and analytical thinking, whilst the right hemisphere shows particular ability with respect to overall perception, and emotional, non-verbal and intuitive thinking (Ames, 1991). Of course, such a dichotomy is over-simplistic, but it is a useful framework in which to consider the neuropsychological differences between men and women detailed above.

Thus, many of the neuropsychological test performance differences between males and females outlined above have been interpreted in terms of cerebral laterality although, as Ames (1991) puts it, 'the two hemispheres function together in both sexes, but appear to differ in the manner in which they do so'.

McGlone (1980) performed a detailed review of the literature on hemispheric laterality, and concluded that, in general, males are more 'lateralized' in terms of their neuropsychological functioning than their female counterparts. Furthermore, the rates of development of the cerebral hemispheres differ between the sexes, with males having a longer period of left hemisphere development (Taylor, 1969); this might account for the particular vulnerability of males to developmental brain insults affecting speech and language (for example, autism). Indeed, the particular vulnerability of the male brain to early insult is evidenced by the fact that, amongst low-birth-weight infants, males are more likely to suffer peri-intraventricular haemorrhage (Amato et al., 1987) and to show longer-term consequences in terms of neuropsychological functioning (Brothwood et al., 1986). The converse of this is that females appear to be relatively protected from early neuro-developmental insult, and the female brain might be more able to accommodate or compensate for any such insult as may occur, than the male brain; the less profound lateralization of functions in the female cortex is presumably of importance in this regard.

Brain structural correlates with the relative sex difference in lateralization of neurocognitive functioning have also been shown. The corpus callosum – the 'bridge' between the hemispheres – has been an obvious focus of interest in this regard. Many studies of the corpus callosum area in males and females are confounded by body size, age and handedness, but Witelson's (1989) elegant work controlled for these factors and she concluded that there are true sex differences in the isthmus of the corpus callosum, with a larger area in females. Thus, Witelson suggests that:

the larger isthmus in (consistently right-handed) females . . . is compatible with the neuropsychological hypothesis of greater bi-hemispheric representation of cognitive functions in females compared with males; it is compatible with the more specific hypothesis of greater bi-hemispheric representation of functions in females for only posterior cortical regions, with females having speech and other praxic functions more focally represented in the left frontal regions; it is compatible with the existence of sex differences in performance on some linguistic and spatial tasks which may be dependent on the temporal and parietal cortices which send fibres through the isthmus.

Ames (1991) has placed these gender differences in an evolutionary context, suggesting that males, as hunters, were evolutionarily advantaged if they exhibited prowess at route finding, and had good visuospatial skills and hand–eye coordination, to facilitate hunting. Females, on the other hand:

lived in a more geographically restricted area and spent time digging up edible plants, handling pots, cooking, and caring for children. These tasks enhance manual dexterity and women might also have become adept at perception of changes in the behaviour and the facial expression of children. Speech 'superiority' in women is less easily explained. It was a relatively late human acquisition. Verbal communication in women may have been accelerated by their close contact with children, which necessitated a greater repertoire of sounds than the shouts and grunts of male hunters.

Whilst this evolutionary perspective might appear over-simplistic, it does serve to introduce a discussion of the evolution of language, as this is a uniquely human attribute, and it is a disturbance of language that is central to many of the symptoms of schizophrenia.

Crow (1994) has extrapolated from findings of gender differences in schizophrenia, and more particularly gender differences in cerebral laterality, to propose a model for schizophrenia as a defect of cerebral lateralization, tied to the development of language. He suggests that: 'From the potential for hemispheric specialisation, by means of a delay in maturation and an increase in brain size, evolved the capacity for a high degree of communication and social interaction, together with diversity in psychological style'. Indeed, he has gone so far as to say that schizophrenia is 'the price [humans] pay for language', and proposed that 'the origins of psychosis are intrinsic and to be sought in the genetic mechanisms associated with the evolution of language'. Furthermore, he hypothesizes that 'a sex difference in the rate of hemispheric differentiation could account for sexual dimorphism for cerebral asymmetry, be relevant to the sex differences in age at onset of psychosis, and provide a clue to the mechanism of these evolutionary developments'. Whilst this view remains speculative, it does point up how the understanding of the mechanisms underlying psychosis can potentially be enhanced through a consideration of gender differences in normal cerebral development and organization, as well as encompassing some of what is known about differences between men and women with schizophrenia.

Behavioural differences between boys and girls

Any interpretation of gender differences in schizophrenia also needs to take account of differences between normal males and females in terms of behaviour. Thus, it is as well to review what is known about differences in the behaviour of boys and girls, for that knowledge can inform consideration of gender differences in behaviour of adults, and particularly, for our purposes, shed light on differences in vulnerability to, and expression of, psychotic illnesses between the sexes.

There has been considerable debate about the extent to which behavioural differences between boys and girls are biologically determined, and to what extent environmental factors influence sexually dichotomous behaviours. Indeed, Earls (1987) has pointed out how two extensive reviews of the subject reached rather different conclusions. Thus, Garai & Scheinfeld (1968) appear to favour innate biological determinants, stating that: 'the male has an innate drive to act upon and transform the environment; and consequently to engage in exciting and challenging investigation of the numerous unfamiliar objects, shapes, and machines'; in contrast, females are 'content to absorb experiences more passively, waiting for stimulation from the environment'. These authors also suggest a difference in socialization between boys and girls: boys tend to be more able to absorb themselves in solitary play, whilst girls 'show a much earlier and greater interest in people, and [their] eagerness to communicate and get along with people leads to earlier and greater verbal fluency'. Thus, these authors suggest innate differences between boys and girls which have profound consequences for the way they interact with the environment and how they perform as social beings.

Maccoby & Jacklin (1980), on the other hand, stress the importance of societal determinants in gender differences in behaviour, suggesting that 'leadership in groups of mature human beings is exercised through persuasion, inspiration, and task competence, and neither sex has an intrinsic advantage in these domains'.

To enlighten this debate, we need to consider those studies which have assessed behavioural differences between boys and girls, and have considered the impact of such differences on later emotional and psychological functioning. In behavioural terms, the epidemiological studies of Richman and colleagues (1982) and of Earls (1987) allow an estimate of prevalence, correlates and course of emotional problems of children from as early as 3 years of age. Both studies showed sex differences – albeit very modest ones – in early childhood, with an excess of overactivity and concentration problems amongst the boys, whilst girls were more likely to exhibit 'several fears'. Of particular interest in the study by Richman et al. was that overactivity and restlessness at 3 years predicted later sociopathy, whilst fearfulness predicted neurotic problems in later childhood. In the study reported by Earls (1987), overactivity and encopresis in early childhood predicted later aggression, delinquency and poor social competence in boys, but for girls there was far less specificity of association between early and later behavioural attributes. Such data suggest that there are early behavioural differences between boys and girls, and that such differences go some way towards explaining sex differences in adult psychopathology; the data also suggest that the developmental trajectories and determination are less clear in girls than boys.

Finally, we turn to a consideration of gender differences in sexual behaviour in humans. Dorner (1977) reported that in rats manipulation of the androgen environment during the critical period of brain development resulted in a tendency to the adoption of sexual behaviour of the opposite gender. The extrapolation to humans is tenuous, but investigation of individuals with congenital adrenal hyperplasia, and those women exposed *in utero* to diethylstilbestrol, appears to support an important neurodevelopmental role for testosterone in the determination of adult sexual behaviour (Pilgrim & Reisert, 1992). Furthermore, evidence from twin studies suggests a genetic component to sexual behaviour (expressly homosexuality), and postmortem studies have found size differences in certain hypothalamic nuclei between individuals of homosexual compared with those of heterosexual persuasion (LeVay, 1991). None of this denies the importance of psychosocial factors in the determination of sexual orientation, but suggests that early biological developmental influences, be they genetic or hormonal, play some part.

Psychiatric differences between boys and girls: a developmental perspective

As we have already pointed out, boys and girls show a differential vulnerability to neurodevelopmental disorders: girls are much less susceptible to disorders such as autism, for example. The explanation for this discrepancy in terms of differential rates of cerebral maturation (expressly, slower development of the left hemisphere in the male fetus) has already been alluded to. However, the finding should be seen in the broader context of a higher risk of prenatal and perinatal death and of mental retardation in males.

Of the early childhood disorders, attention deficit hyperactivity disorder (ADHD) is also far less prevalent in girls than boys. Indeed, the population-based Ontario Child Mental Health Survey found a prevalence of ADHD of 12.7% in boys aged 4–11 years, whilst no cases were found amongst girls at any age. Whether this differential vulnerability between the sexes is determined by the same factors as those operating in mental retardation and autism is not clear.

By school age, and into adolescence, differences between girls and boys in terms of psychiatric morbidity become more emphatic. The Ontario Child Mental Health Survey, for example, reported that conduct disorder was more common in boys and neurosis and somatization more common in girls across all ages from 4 to 16 years.

These gender differences persist into adulthood. For example, the population-based Epidemiological Catchment Area Study in the US (Robins et al., 1984) found that males exceeded females in rates of suicide, antisocial personality disorder and alcoholism, whilst females were more vulnerable to anxiety, depression and somatization.

Again, these gender differences in vulnerability to psychiatric illness need to be considered in any explanatory model of gender differences in psychosis.

The aging brain

We have outlined a number of domains where the brains and neuro-psychological functioning of males and females appear to deviate from each other from early in development. To counterpose this literature, there is also evidence that male and female brains age differently (Castle, 1999).

It is well established in neuropathological studies that the human brain shows age-related decreases in weight and volume and a loss of cortical neurones. More recently, neuroimaging studies have allowed systematic consideration of age-related changes in specific cortical regions and in subcortical structures. For example, Jernigan et al. (1991) performed magnetic resonance imaging (MRI) scans on 55 individuals (21 female) with no history of dementia, ranging in age from 30 to 79 years (mean 53.8; SD 14.1). They found significant age-related decreases in the volume of the caudate nucleus and in anterior diencephalic structures, whilst there was little noticeable change in thalamic volume. There were also volume reductions in cortical grey matter, which were most marked in association with cortex and mesial temporal lobe structures; it appeared that anterior cingulate cortex was relatively spared.

Murphy and colleagues (1996) conducted a study specifically to assess gender differences in age-related brain changes. These investigators performed MRI scans on 69 healthy right-handed individuals (34 female) divided into two age groups, namely 20–35 years and 60–85 years. They found that, whilst male brains showed greater age-related loss of whole-brain and frontal and temporal lobe volume than their female counterparts, females showed more extensive volume loss with age in the parietal lobe and hippocampus. There were also differences in right–left asymmetry with age between men and women; the left hemisphere was particularly affected in females.

A study of brain metabolism, measured by positron emission tomography (PET), also showed a differential effect of age in men and women (Murphy et al., 1996). Thus, women showed more age-related metabolic decline in thalamus and hippocampus than their male counterparts; the hippocampal metabolism in females became less than in males around the age of 70 years.

Given the involvement of dopaminergic pathways in the pathogenesis of psychotic symptoms, it is worth considering the effect of age on the dopamine system. Wong et al. (1984) reported loss of D_2 receptors in caudate, putamen and frontal cortex in men and women aged 19–73 years. The rate and pattern of loss differed between the sexes: males showed an exponential decline in D_2 receptors, whilst for females the decline was essentially linear. A more recent study of dopamine D_2 receptor density in 33 men and 21 women (age 19–82 years; mean 40.2; SD 16.7), also using PET, confirmed the sex differential, with men showing a rate of decline in D_2 receptors twice that of women (Pohjalainen et al., 1998). The decline in D_2 receptor density begins at a relatively young age (under 20 years, and earlier for males than females). The cross-over in rate of decline between men and women occurs at around the age of 30 years (extrapolated from figures presented in Wong et al., 1984). Thus, males start with a relative excess of D_2 receptors in comparison to women, but lose them earlier and more rapidly, such that in later life it is females who have a relative excess of these receptors.

Conclusions

This chapter has reviewed gender differences in brain development and organization and outlined behavioural and neuropsychological differences between males and females. It has also looked at differential susceptibilities of boys and girls to brain insult, as well as to behavioural and emotional disorders, and established links with gender differences in these parameters in adults. Finally, it has outlined the established gender differences in the aging brain. We believe that any consideration of gender differences in psychosis must take into account this broad context.

Acknowledgements

The author is most grateful to Professors Lynn DeLisi (New York) and Frances Ames (Cape Town) for their suggestions and comments on earlier drafts of this chapter.

REFERENCES

Amato, M., Howald H. & von Muralt, G. (1987). Fetal sex and distribution of peri-ventricular hemorrhage in preterm infants. *Eur. Neurol.,* **27**, 20–3.

Ames F.R. (1991). Sex and the brain. *S. Afr. Med. J.,* **80**, 150–2.

Berenbaum S.A. & Hines, M. (1992). Early androgens are related to childhood sex-typed toy preferences. *Psychol. Sci.*, **3**, 203–6.

Breedlove, S.M. (1994). Sexual differentiation of the human nervous system. *Annu. Rev. Psychol.*, **45**, 389–418.

Brothwood, M., Wolke, D., Gamsu, H., Benson, J. & Cooper, D. (1986). Prognosis of the very low birthweight baby in relation to gender. *Arch. Dis. Child.*, **61**, 559–64.

Castle, D.J. (1999). Gender and age at onset in schizophrenia. In *Late Onset Schizophrenia*, ed. R. Howard, P. Rabins & D. Castle, pp. 147–64. Hampshire: Wrightson Biomedical.

Crow, T.J. (1994). Syndromes of schizophrenia. *Br. J. Psychiatry*, **165**, 721–7.

Diamond, M. (1989). Sex and the cerebral cortex. *Biol. Psychiatry*, **25**, 823–5.

Dorner, G. (1977). Hormone dependent differentiation, maturation and function of the brain and sexual behaviour. *Endokrinologie*, **69**, 306–20.

Earls, F. (1987). Sex differences in psychiatric disorders: origins and developmental influences. *Psychiatr. Dev.*, **1**, 1–23.

Finegan, J., Bartelman, B. & Wong, P.Y. (1988). A window for the study of prenatal sex hormone influences on postnatal development. *J. Genet. Psychol.*, **150**, 101–12.

Garai, J. & Scheinfeld, A. (1968). Sex differences in mental and behavioural traits. *Genet. Psychol. Monogr.*, **77**, 169–299.

Gorski, R.A., Harlan, R.E., Jacobsen, C.D., Shryne, J.E. & Southam, A.M. (1980). Evidence for the existence of a sexually dimorphic nucleus in the preoptic region of the rat. *J. Comp. Neurol.*, **193**, 529–39.

Haug, H. (1984). Macroscopic and microscopic morphometry of the human brain and cortex. A survey in the light of new results. *Brain Pathol.*, **1**, 123–49.

Hier, D.B. & Crowley, W.F. (1982). Spatial ability in androgen-deficient men. *N. Engl. J. Med.*, **306**, 1202–5.

Hines, M. (1982). Prenatal gonadal hormones and sex differences in human behaviour. *Psychol. Bull.*, **92**, 56–80.

Jernigan, T.L., Archibald, S.L., Berhow, M.T., Sowell, E.R., Foster, D.S. & Hesselink, J.R. (1991). Cerebral structure on MRI: Part 1: Localisation of age-related changes. *Biol. Psychiatry*, **29**, 55–67.

Kimura, D. (1992). Sex differences in the brain. *Sci. Am.*, **267**, 118–25.

LeVay, S. (1991). A difference in hypothalamic structure between heterosexual and homosexual men. *Science*, **253**, 1034–7.

Maccoby, E.E. & Jacklin, C.N. (1980). Psychological sex differences. In *Scientific Foundations of Developmental Psychiatry*, ed. M. Rutter, pp. 92–100. London: Heinemann Medical.

McGee, M.G. (1982). Spatial abilities: the influence of genetic factors. In *Spatial Orientation: Developments and Physiological Bases*, ed. M. Potegal, pp. 199–222. New York: Academic Press.

McGlone, J. (1980). Sex differences in human brain asymmetry: a critical survey. Behav. Brain Sci., **3**, 215–63.

Murphy, D.G.M., DeCarli, C., McIntosh, A.R. et al. (1996). Sex differences in human brain morphometry and meabolism: an *in-vivo* quantitative magnetic resonance imaging and positron emission tomography study on the effect of aging. *Arch. Gen. Psychiatry*, **53**, 585–94.

Nottenbohm, F. & Arnold, A.P. (1976). Sexual dimorphism in vocal control areas of the songbird brain. *Science*, **194**, 211–13.

Phoenix, C.H., Goy, R.W., Gerall, A.A. & Young, W.C. (1959). Organising action of prenatally administered testosterone propionate on the tissues mediating mating behaviour in the female guinea pig. *Endocrinology*, **65**, 369–82.

Pilgrim, Ch. & Reisert, I. (1992). Differences between male and female brains – developmental mechanisms and implications. *Horm. Metab. Res.*, **24**, 353–9.

Pohjalainen, T., Rinne, J.O., Nagren, K., Syvalahti, E. & Hietala, J. (1998). Sex differences in the striatal dopamine D_2 receptor binding *in vivo*. *Am. J. Psychiatry*, **155**, 768–73.

Reisert, I. & Pilgrim, Ch. (1991). Sexual differentiation of monoaminergic neurons – genetic or epigenetic? *Trends Neurosci.*, **14**, 468–73.

Reite, M., Sheeder, J., Teale, P. et al. (1997). Magnetic source imaging evidence of sex differences in cerebral lateralisation in schizophrenia. *Arch. Gen. Psychiatry*, **54**: 433–40.

Resnick, S.M., Berenbaum, S.A., Gottesman II & Bouchard, T.J. (1986). Early hormonal influences on cognitive functioning in congenital adrenal hyperplasia. *Dev. Psychol.*, **22**. 191–8.

Richman, N., Stevenson, J. & Graham, P. (1982). *Preschool to School: A Behavioural Study*. London: Academic Press.

Robins, L.N., Helzer, J.E., Weissman, M.M. et al. (1984). Lifetime prevalence of specific psychiatric disorders in three sites. *Arch. Gen. Psychiatry*, **41**, 157–61.

Schwartz, C.E. (1993). X-linked mental retardation: in pursuit of a gene map. *Am. J. Hum. Genet.*, **52**: 1025–31.

Swaab, D.F. & Fliers, E. (1985). A sexually dimorphic nucleus in the human brain. *Science*, **228**, 1112–15.

Taylor, D.C. (1969). Differential rates of cerebral maturation between sexes and between hemispheres. *Lancet*, **ii**: 140–2.

Wada, J.A., Clarke, R. & Hamm, A. (1975). Cerebral hemispheric asymmetry in humans. *Arch. Neurol.*, 32, 239–46.

Witelson, S.F. (1989). Hand and sex differences in the isthmus and genu of the human corpus callosum. *Brain*, **112**, 799–835.

Wong, D.F., Wagner, H.N., Dannals, R.F. et al. (1984). Effects of age on dopamine and serotonin receptors measured by positron emission tomography in the living human brain. *Science*, **226**: 1393–6.

3

Women and schizophrenia: an epidemiological perspective

David J. Castle

There have been a number of recent comprehensive reviews of gender differences in the epidemiology of schizophrenia and related disorders (Angermeyer & Kuhn, 1988; Lewine, 1988; Goldstein, 1995a; Piccinelli & Gomez Homen, 1997). This chapter does not seek to recapitulate these reviews, but rather focuses on some of the more controversial and novel findings, and sets these findings in a interpretative framework.

Are females less prone to schizophrenia?

The starting point for a discussion about the epidemiology of schizophrenia in women is to establish whether women are more or less prone than men to the manifestation of the disorder. This is an important issue, as any major gender disparity in rates of illness would suggest a particular vulnerability of one of the sexes to the disorder.

Conventional wisdom has it that both men and women carry around a 1% lifetime risk of schizophrenia; that is, that both sexes are equally prone. But this bland conclusion hides a number of caveats, including the fact that the gender ratio is markedly affected by the diagnostic criteria applied. Readers will be aware of the lack of consistency amongst clinicians and researchers as to what is subsumed under the label 'schizophrenia'. The disproportionate ease with which the label could be applied in the US, compared to the UK, in the 1970s, was made clear by the landmark US/UK diagnostic project (Cooper et al., 1972) which established that most discrepancy in rates of schizophrenia on opposite sides of the Atlantic was accounted for by differences in diagnostic habit.

The US/UK diagnostic project contributed to the establishment of operationalized criteria for schizophrenia, a move which, whilst enhancing reliability of diagnosis, lulled researchers into a false sense of security about the validity of the schizophrenia concept. Indeed, there remains no objective validating sign, symptom, or test which makes the diagnosis, and different sets of diagnostic criteria include or exclude different groups of patients from the diagnosis. For example, the restrictive criteria of Feighner and colleagues (1972) include loadings for an onset of illness before age 40 years, and a family history of schizophrenia, and insist on at least 6 months' duration of illness. The Research Diagnostic Criteria (RDC) of Spitzer and colleagues (1978) are far more liberal, allowing a diagnosis after only 2 weeks of illness, and removing the age-at-onset and family history loadings.

Whilst this discussion may seem trivial, it is in fact vital in the consideration of gender differences in schizophrenia, as different sets of diagnostic criteria, when applied to the same group of men and women with psychotic disorders, diagnose different proportions of males and females as having schizophrenia. An illustration of this is provided in Table 3.1, which shows female-to-male ratios according to a number of different sets of diagnostic criteria, applied to an incident sample of patients with a broad range of non-affective psychotic presentations (Castle et al., 1993). The effect of the different diagnostic criteria on the gender ratio is profound. Thus, the restrictive Feighner criteria diagnose far more males than females as having schizophrenia, whilst application of the RDC results in a gender ratio of close to unity.

So, are both sexes in fact equally susceptible to schizophrenia? In the light of the above discussion, the question loses meaning, and can only be responded to by asking what is meant by the diagnostic label 'schizophrenia'. It seems clear that, if a severe early-onset type of illness is considered, there is a male excess. On the other hand, inclusion of later-onset 'milder' cases redresses this gender imbalance. What remains unclarified is whether the later-onset, female-preponderant group have essentially the same disorder as their early-onset counterparts, but with a delayed onset, or whether they represent a separate subtype of disorder. To take forward this theme, we turn now to an appraisal of the literature on gender and age at onset in schizophrenia.

Table 3.1. Gender ratio according to different sets of diagnostic criteria for schizophrenia

Diagnostic criteria	Incidence rate per 100 000 per year		Female : male ratio
	Females	Males	
ICD-9 (schizophrenia and related disorders)			
Onset <45 years	17.8	25.2	0.71 : 1
Onset >45 years	17.1	10.4	1.64 : 1
All ages at onset	17.6	19.2	0.92 : 1
RDC			
Onset <45 years	10.4	16.4	0.63 : 1
Onset >45 years	14.3	8.7	1.64 : 1
All ages at onset	11.9	13.7	0.87 : 1
DSM-IIIR			
Onset <45 years	5.2	11.1	0.47 : 1
Onset >45 years	9.0	5.2	1.73 : 1
All ages at onset	6.7	9.0	0.74 : 1
DSM-III			
Onset <45 years	6.3	13.9	0.45 : 1
Feighner criteria			
Onset <40 years	6.0	14.8	0.41 : 1

From Castle et al., 1993.

A later onset of schizophrenia in females?

It is almost universally accepted that schizophrenia first manifests at a later mean age in females than males. Table 3.2 presents a number of studies from different settings with different designs, and applying different sets of diagnostic criteria, which attest to this. An obvious question is whether this is an artefact due to differences in help-seeking behaviour between males and females with schizophrenia. For example, some authors have suggested that the greater likelihood of aggression in males with schizophrenia would bring them to the attention of services earlier than their female counterparts. Conversely, it has been suggested that females with schizophrenia are

Table 3.2. Gender differences in age at onset of schizophrenia (selected studies only)

Author	Country	Age range (years)	Diagnostic criteria	Definition of onset	Mean age at onset (years) Female	Mean age at onset (years) Male
Munk-Jørgensen (1986)	Denmark	No age limit	ICD-8	First admission	33.7	27.4
Hafner et al. (1993)	Germany	12–59	ICD-9	First sign of mental disorder	27.5	24.3
				First psychotic symptoms	30.6	26.5
				First acute episode	31.7	27.8
Castle et al. (1993)	UK	16+	ICD-9, schizophrenia and related disorders	First contact with psychiatric services	41.1	31.2
Susser & Wanderling (1994)	Developing countries (India, Colombia, Nigeria)	15–54	ICD-9	First contact with treating agency	25.7	23.0
	Developed countries (Denmark, Ireland, Russia, Japan, UK, USA, Czech Republic)	15–54	ICD-9	First contact with treating agency	30.7	26.0
Faraone et al. (1994)	USA	No age limit	DSM-III	First psychotic symptoms	31.1	26.2
Szymanski et al. (1995)	USA	16–40	RDC	First psychotic symptoms	24.0	21.0
				First hospitalization	24.0	22.0

more likely to be protected by their families, and that social role expectations would make them less likely than males to come to the attention of psychiatric services. Whilst such factors may play a role, it appears that overall it cannot account for the extent of the age differential between the sexes. The ABC Study of Hafner and colleagues (1993; see Table 3.2) is instructive in this regard. These authors went to great pains to determine onset of illness, and compared males and females according to three definitions of onset: age at first sign of mental disorder, age at first psychotic symptoms and age at first acute episode of illness. Whichever definition of onset was used, females had a later onset than males; furthermore, the mean lag between onset and hospitalization was much the same for both sexes.

Another way of looking at this issue is that a later onset of illness in females has been found in a diversity of settings. The World Health Organization Ten Country Study (Jablensky et al., 1992), for example, determined first episodes of schizophrenia in a wide variety of urban and rural settings (Table 3.2), and a later mean onset in females was reported for all sites (Hambrecht et al., 1992). Thus, it is unlikely that either help-seeking behaviour or service delivery factors can explain away findings of a later onset of illness in females.

Another potential problem in studies of gender differences in onset of schizophrenia lies in a failure to control for gender differences in the base population, including the fact that women tend to live longer than men, and that they are less likely to die young than are their male counterparts. Faraone and colleagues (1994) examined gender differences in age at onset of schizophrenia, controlling for these parameters. The observed later onset of schizophrenia in women could not be explained away by the longevity of women in the general population, nor by differential mortality between the sexes.

If we accept that females do tend to have a later onset of illness than males, we need to consider factors which might confound this finding; that is, factors associated with both a later onset of illness as well as with being female. Of the factors reportedly associated with a later onset of illness, a negative family history of schizophrenia (Sham et al., 1994; Alda et al., 1996), a good developmental trajectory (Foerster et al., 1991; Jablensky & Cole, 1997) and a negative history for those pregnancy and birth complications implicated in the aetiogenesis of schizophrenia (Verdoux et al., 1997) are the most robust. Of these, the good premorbid course and negative history of pregnancy and birth complications are also more characteristic of females, than males, with schizophrenia. On the other hand, a positive family history of schizophrenia has been found to be more common in females, than males, with schizophrenia (Goldstein, 1995b). It is possible that females require more aetiological 'hits' before they manifest schizophrenia at an early age than do their male counterparts, and that one of these 'hits' is genetic (as evidenced by a family loading for the illness). Alternatively, females may be less prone than males to non-genetic aetiological factors in schizophrenia; this latter hypothesis would tally with the higher risk of pregnancy and birth complications in males with schizophrenia, expressly those with an early illness onset. Another issue which has only recently been systematically addressed is that in highly familial samples of schizophrenia patients the sex differential at age at onset all but disappears (Alda et al., 1996).

Turning to social confounding factors, it has been shown that being married tends to protect against an early onset of illness. It is also clear that females are more likely than males to be married at the time of onset of illness. Few studies have formally evaluated whether marital status can explain away the finding of a later onset of illness in females. However, Jablensky & Cole (1997) examined this issue in a sample of 653 women and 778 men, ascertained as part of the World Health Organization's Ten Country Study. Generalized linear modelling was used to estimate the unconfounded contributions of premorbid personality, family history of schizophrenia and marital status to age at onset in females and males. Whilst females did show a later mean onset than males (28.94 years vs. 25.36 years for males; $p < 0.0001$), much of this difference was accounted for by marital status (being married was associated with a later onset) and premorbid personality disorder (associated with an early onset of illness). A positive family history of schizophrenia exhibited a weaker effect (associated with early illness onset). These authors concluded that being married tended of itself to delay onset of illness, and that this effect was most marked for males.

Age-at-onset distribution curves for males and females

The discussion above has focused on mean age at onset of illness in males and females. However, it should be noted that the reliance on means, and a comparison of means, is misleading and statistically indefensible, in that age-at-onset distribution curves for men and women with schizophrenia are complex and not unimodal. Furthermore, the onset distribution curves for males and females are not isomorphic; that is, it is not as though the curve for females is simply shifted to the right. For example, the ABC Study of Hafner and colleagues (1993) in Mannheim, Germany, reported males to show a dramatic early peak of onset, with a monotonous decline after the age of around 30; females, on the other hand, showed a lesser early peak, and a later peak in the 40s. Data from the WHO Ten Country Study also reveal the differences in the shape of the distributions between the sexes. Hambrecht and colleagues (1992) pooled these data and showed that the distributions were very similar to the Mannheim data.

The reported studies above all suffer from one major drawback with respect to a comparison of males and females with schizophrenia, namely that they imposed an age cut-off. For example, the ABC study did not include patients with an onset over the age of 59 years, whilst the Ten Country Study only looked at patients with an onset before 55 years of age. The problem with excluding patients with a very late onset of illness (i.e. after 55 or 60 years) lies in that group having a very marked preponderance of females. Indeed, Table 3.3 shows a number of studies of patients with late- and very-late-onset schizophrenia, which employed different sampling frames, and applied different sets of diagnostic criteria, but which all had a high female-to-male ratio. This excess of females in late-onset schizophrenia is not merely a reflection of the relative longevity in females; indeed, the incidence rate ratios in the Camberwell Register study (Castle *et al.*, 1993; Table 3.3) are based on actual population-determined rates, and do not rely merely on relative numbers of women and men.

Thus, a true appraisal of differences in age-at-onset distribution between the sexes can only be made with those few studies which have not imposed an arbitrary age cut-off. One such study is the Camberwell Register study, cited above and in Table 3.3. In essence, this study included all patients with a non-affective non-organic psychotic disorder, presenting for the first time

Table 3.3. Selected series of late-onset schizophrenia patients reporting gender ratio

Author	No. of cases	Ascertainment method	Diagnosis	Age (years)	Ratio female : male
Kay (1963)	57	Hospital admissions	Late paraphrenia[a]	>60	5.3 : 1
Herbert & Jacobsen (1967)	47	Hospital admissions	Systematized delusion ± hallucinations; not demented	>65	22.5 : 1
Huber et al. (1975)	644	Hospital admissions	Late-onset schizophrenia; not organic	>40	1.8 : 1
Bland (1977)	6064	First admissions	ICD-8 schizophrenia	>40	1.6 : 1
Blessed & Wilson (1982)	320	Hospital admissions	Late paraphrenia[a]	>65	6 : 1
Grahame (1984)	25	Consecutive referrals	Late paraphrenia[a]	>60	3.2 : 1
Rabins et al. (1984)	35	Hospital admissions	Persistent delusional state; absence of mood or cognitive disorder	Onset >40	10.7 : 1
Jørgensen & Munk-Jørgensen (1985)	106	First admissions	ICD-8 schizophrenia, paranoid state, reactive psychosis, other psychoses	>60	2.2 : 1
Holden (1987)	37	Case register	Late paraphrenia[a] (13 cases considered 'organic' at follow-up)	>60	7 : 1 to 3 : 1[b]
Castle & Murray (1993)	477	Case register	ICD-9 schizophrenia and related disorders, paraphrenia, atypical psychoses	>60	4.4 : 1
Almeida et al. (1995)	47	Referrals from a number of psychiatric settings	Late paraphrenia[a]	>65	9 : 1

[a] Akin to Roth's (1955) criteria.
[b] Dependent on whether 'organic' cases are included.
Reproduced with permission from Castle (1999).

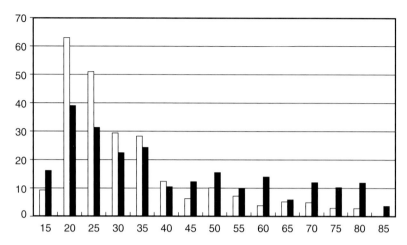

Figure 3.1   Distribution of age at onset of schizophrenia for males (open columns) and females (filled columns). Reproduced with permission from Castle (1999).

to the psychiatric services of Camberwell, south-east London between the years 1965 and 1984. The distribution curves for males and females are shown in Figure 3.1. It will be noted that there are at least three peaks of onset, and that males and females are disproportionately distributed with respect to these onset peaks. Thus, the early-onset peak shows a marked excess of males; the middle-onset peak is female-preponderant; and the very-late-onset peak is almost exclusive to females.

A more sophisticated way of looking at these data is to perform an admixture analysis, which allows a statistical exploration of the distributions. In the Camberwell data, this approach revealed a best-fit explanation for the male distribution as encompassing two onset peaks, with modal onsets of 21.4 and 39.2 years, respectively. For females, on the other hand, there were three peaks, with modes at 22.4, 36.6 and 61.5 years (Castle et al., 1998).

In a separate study, McLachlan and colleagues (1998) obtained first admission data from the Queensland (Australia) Mental Health Register and fitted mixture models to the data. For those cases meeting ICD 8/9 criteria for schizophrenia ($n = 7651$), a three-component model, with different mean ages of onset, best fitted the distribution for both sexes, but the proportion of males and females in each component was different. Thus, 20% of females, compared to 29% of males, were included in the first component (mean age at onset 22 years for both sexes), whilst 47% of females and only 32% of males were in the third component (mean age at onset 52 years for females and 48 years for males).

Explanatory hypotheses

The cumulation of the epidemiological evidence outlined in this chapter points to the following:

1 Females are less likely than males to meet stringent diagnostic criteria for schizophrenia.
2 Females tend to manifest the illness for the first time at a later age than males, and this is not merely an artefact due to psychosocial differences between men and women.
3 The onset curves for males and females are not isomorphic.

How can these disparate findings be accounted for in a single explanatory hypothesis? One suggestion has been that something about being female both delays the onset and ameliorates the symptoms of schizophrenia. The most popular candidate is estrogen. This hypothesis has merit, as is detailed in Chapter 5. However, it is difficult to conceive how estrogen alone can explain the complexity of the age-at-onset distribution curves; for example, why should prepubescent schizophrenia be more common in males, and how can estrogen withdrawal account for the male peak (albeit smaller than that for females) in the mid-40s; and how can estrogen withdrawal account for the massive female excess amongst very-late-onset patients? Furthermore, how can the estrogen protection hypothesis be compatible with the finding that, in highly familial samples, males and females tend not to show the usual difference in age at onset of schizophrenia?

An alternative approach is an explanatory model based on subtypes of schizophrenia, with different mean ages at onset, and which affect males and females differentially. This approach has been articulated elsewhere (Castle & Murray, 1991; Murray et al., 1992; Castle et al., 1994; Sham et al., 1996). In brief, it has been proposed that gender differences in brain development, organization and aging, as outlined in Chapter 2, may result, in part at least, in a differential vulnerability of females and males to different subtypes of schizophrenia. For example, the relatively slower development of the left hemisphere in the male brain – a result of testosterone (see Chapter 2) – could explain male vulnerability to neurodevelopmental disorders in general, and to a neurodevelopmental subtype of schizophrenia in particular. It is not that females are spared from this form of the disorder, merely that they are less prone to it. Furthermore, if females do present with an early-onset neurodevelopmental type of schizophrenia, it would be compatible with this hypothesis that they would have a greater number of aetiological 'hits' than their male counterparts. This might explain the greater family loading for schizophrenia in female, compared with male, probands with schizophrenia, as well as the association between early onset and familial loading. It is not the case that a neurodevelopmental model presupposes a non-genetic causation; indeed, it has been suggested that 'the genetics of schizophrenia is the genetics of neurodevelopment' (Jones & Murray, 1991).

At the other extreme of life, the greater female vulnerability to the first manifestation of a schizophrenia-like illness in very late life (late paraphrenia; Table 3.3) may be a reflection of changes in degenerative trajectories between female and male brains (Castle, 1999). Furthermore, the rate of loss of brain dopamine D_2 receptors differs between the sexes, such that males start with a higher density of receptors, but lose them faster than females (see Chapter 2). The net result is that females in later life have a relative excess of D_2 receptors and this might, in part at least, explain their vulnerability to the first onset of schizophrenia in late life, as well as their particular propensity to the development of tardive dyskinesia, thought to be due to dopamine receptor supersensitivity (see Chapter 8).

In middle life, the female schizophrenia excess is more difficult to explain. It is possible that estrogen withdrawal at menopause plays some role here, with the caveats listed above. It may also be that some cases of mid-life-onset schizophrenia in fact have aetiological links with affective disorders which are known to affect females more than males (reviewed by Piccinelli & Gomez Homen, 1997). This proposal is supported by the finding of a higher rate of affective symptoms amongst later-onset females with schizophrenia (see Chapter 4), as well as the marked excess of females amongst patients with so-called cycloid psychoses, thought to be aetiologically linked with affective psychoses, but which present cross-sectionally with psychotic symptoms typical of schizophrenia (Cutting et al., 1978). A further consideration is the marked female preponderance amongst those individuals who present with so-called acute remitting psychosis, where a good long-term outcome is usual (Susser & Wanderling, 1994).

In an attempt to subtype schizophrenia based on gender, we (Castle et al., 1994; Sham et al., 1996) found reasonably robust evidence for an early-onset male preponderant neurodevelopmental form of illness. A later-onset type, exclusive to females, and which showed many affective features and a family loading for affective disorders, went some way towards explaining the female excess in mid-life-onset disorder. There was also a larger mid-life subtype, with the features of the paranoid subtype of schizophrenia described by Tsuang & Winokur (1974). This subtype appeared to affect the sexes equally.

Conclusions

The data presented in this chapter, of a relative paucity of stringently defined schizophrenia amongst women, as well as the tendency to a later onset of illness in women compared with men, lend some of the most compelling evidence of a true difference between the sexes to the group of disorders currently subsumed under the label 'schizophrenia'. One attempt to understand these differences lies in the suggestion that males and females are differentially vulnerable to relatively distinct subtypes of schizophrenia. However, these gender differences in terms of symptom expression, as well as developmental trajectory, must be seen in the context of the broader literature on gender differences in vulnerabilty to, and expression of, mental disorders (see Chapters 2 and 4).

REFERENCES

Alda, M., Ahrens, B., Lit, W. et al. (1996). Age of onset in familial and sporadic schizophrenia. *Acta Psychiatr. Scand.,* **93**, 447–50.

Almeida, O.P., Howard, R.J., Levy, R. & David, A.S. (1995). Cognitive and clinical diversity in psychotic states arising in late life (late paraphrenia). *Psychol. Med.,* **25**, 699–714.

Angermeyer, M.C. & Kuhn, L. (1988). Gender differences in age at onset of schizophrenia: an overview. *Eur. Arch. Psychiatry Neurol. Sci.,* **237**, 351–64.

Bland, R.C. (1977). Demographic aspects of functional psychoses in Canada. *Acta Psychiatr. Scand.*, **55**, 369–80.

Blessed, G. & Wilson, I.D. (1982). The contemporary natural history of mental disorder in old age. *Br. J. Psychiatry*, **141**, 59–67.

Castle, D.J. (1999). Gender and age at onset in schizophrenia. In *Late Onset Schizophrenia* ed. R. Howard, P.V. Rabins & D. Castle, pp. 147–64. Hampshire: Wrightson Biomedical.

Castle, D.J. & Murray, R.M. (1991). The neurodevelopmental basis of gender differences in schizophrenia. *Psychol. Med.*, **21**, 565–75.

Castle, D.J. & Murray, R.M. (1993). The epidemiology of late onset schizophrenia. *Schizophr. Bull.*, **19**, 691–700.

Castle, D.J., Wessely, S. & Murray, R.M. (1993). Sex and schizophrenia: effects of diagnostic stringency, and association with premorbid variables. *Br. J. Psychiatry*, **162**, 658–64.

Castle, D.J., Sham, P., Wessely, S. & Murray, R.M. (1994). The subtyping of schizophrenia in men and women: A latent class analysis. *Psychol. Med.*, **24**, 41–51.

Castle, D.J., Sham, P. & Murray, R.M. (1998). Differences in ages of onset in males and females with schizophrenia. *Schizophr. Res.*, **33**, 179–83.

Cooper, J.E., Kendell, R.E., Gurland, B.J., Sharp, L., Copeland, J.R.M. & Simon, R. (1972). *Psychiatric Diagnosis in New York and London: Maudsley Monograph No. 20.* London: Oxford University Press.

Cutting, J.C., Clare, A.W. & Mann, A.H. (1978). Cycloid psychosis: investigation of diagnostic concept. *Psychol. Med.*, **8**, 637–48.

Faraone, S.V., Chen, W.J., Goldstein, J.M. & Tsuang, M.T. (1994). Gender differences in age at onset of schizophrenia. *Br. J. Psychiatry*, **164**, 625–9.

Feighner, J.P., Robins, E., Guze, S.B., Woodruff, R., Winokur, G. & Munoz, R. (1972). Diagnostic criteria for use in psychiatric research. *Arch. Gen. Psychiatry*, **26**, 57–63.

Foerster, A., Lewis, S.W., Owen, M.J. & Murray, R.M. (1991). Premorbid personality in psychosis: Effects of sex and diagnosis. *Br. J. Psychiatry*, **158**, 171–6.

Goldstein, J.M. (1995a). The impact of gender on understanding the epidemiology of schizophrenia. In *Gender and Psychopathology*, ed. MV Seeman, pp. 159–99. Washington DC: American Psychiatric Press.

Goldstein, J.M. (1995b). Gender and the familial transmission of schizophrenia. In *Gender and Psychopathology*, ed. MV Seeman, pp. 201–26. Washington DC: American Psychiatric Press.

Grahame, P.S. (1984). Schizophrenia in late life (late paraphrenia). *Br. J. Psychiatry*, **145**, 493–5.

Hafner, H., Riecher-Rossler, A., an der Heiden, W., Maurer, K., Fatkenheuer, B. and Loffler, W. (1993). Generating and testing a causal explanation of the gender difference in age at first onset of schizophrenia. *Psychol. Med.*, **23**, 925–40.

Hambrecht, M., Maurer, K., Hafner, H. & Sartorius, N. (1992). Transnational stability of gender differences in schizophrenia. *Eur. Arch. Schizophr. Neurol. Sci.*, **242**, 6–12.

Herbert, M.E. & Jacobsen, S. (1967). Late paraphrenia. *Br. J. Psychiatry*, **113**, 461–9.

Holden, N.L. (1987). Late paraphrenia or the paraphrenias? A descriptive study with 10-year follow up. *Br. J. Psychiatry*, **150**, 635–9.

Huber, G., Gross, G. & Schuttler, R. (1975). Spatzschizophrenie. *Arch. Psychiatr. Nervenkrankh*, **221**, 53–66.

Jablensky, A. & Cole, S. (1997). Is the earlier age at onset of schizophrenia in males a confounded finding? Results from a cross-cultural investigation. *Br. J. Psychiatry*, **170**, 234–40.

Jablensky, A., Sartorius, N., Ernberg, G. et al. (1992). *Schizophrenia: Manifestations, Incidence and Course in Different Cultures. A World Health Organisation Ten-Country Study. Psychological Medicine Monograph 20.* Cambridge: Cambridge University Press.

Jones, P.B., Murray, R.M. (1991). The genetics of schizophrenia is the genetics of neurodevelopment. *Br. J. Psychiatry*, **168**, 615–23.

Jørgensen P. & Munk-Jørgensen, P. (1985). Paranoid psychoses in the elderly. *Acta Psychiatr. Scand.*, **72**, 358–63.

Kay, D.W.K. (1963). Late paraphrenia and its bearing on the aetiology of schizophrenia. *Acta Psychiatr. Scand.*, **39**, 159–69.

Lewine, R.J. (1988). Gender and schizophrenia. In *Handbook of Schizophrenia*, vol. 3, ed. HA Nasrallah. Amsterdam: Elsevier.

McLachlan, G., Welham J. & McGrath J. (1998). Heterogeneity in schizophrenia: a mixture model analysis based on age-of-onset, gender and diagnosis. *Schizophr. Res.*, **29**, 25.

Munk-Jørgensen, P. (1986). Schizophrenia in Denmark. Incidence and utilisation of psychiatric institutions. *Acta Psychiatr. Scand.*, **73**, 172–80.

Murray, R.M., O'Callaghan, E., Castle, D.J. & Lewis, S.W. (1992). A neurodevelopmental approach to the classification of schizophrenia. *Schizophr. Bull.*, **18**, 319–22.

Piccinelli, M. & Gomez Homen, F. (1997). *Gender Differences in the Epidemiology of Affective Disorders and Schizophrenia.* Geneva: World Health Organization.

Rabins, P., Paulker, S. & Thomas, J. (1984). Can schizophrenia begin after age 44? *Compr. Psychiatry*, **25**, 290–3.

Roth, M. (1955). The natural history of mental disorder in old age. *J. Ment. Sci.*, **101**, 281–301.

Sham, P.C., Jones, P., Russell, A. et al. (1994). Age at onset, sex, and familial psychiatric history in schizophrenia. *Br. J. Psychiatry*, **165**, 466–73.

Sham, P., Castle, D.J., Wessely, S., Farmer, A. & Murray, R.M. (1996). Further exploration of a latent class typology of schizophrenia. *Schizophr. Res.*, **20**, 105–15.

Spitzer, R., Endicott, J. & Robins, E. (1978). Research Diagnostic Criteria (RDC):

rationale and reliability. *Arch. Gen. Psychiatry*, **35**, 773–82.

Susser, E. & Wanderling, J. (1994). Epidemiology of acute remitting psychosis vs. schizophrenia. *Arch. Gen. Psychiatry*, **51**, 294–301.

Szymanski, S., Lieberman, J.A., Alvir, J.M. et al. (1995). Gender differences in onset of illness, treatment response, course, and biological indexes in first-episode schizophrenic patients. *Am. J. Psychiatry*, **152**, 698–703.

Tsuang, M.T. & Winokur, G. (1974). Criteria for subtyping schizophrenia: clinical differentiation of hebephrenic and paranoid schizophrenia. *Arch. Gen. Psychiatry*, **31**, 43–7.

Verdoux, H., Geddes, J.R., Takei, N. et al. (1997). Obstetric complications and age at onset of schizophrenia: an international meta analysis of individual patient data. *Am. J. Psychiatry*, **154**, 1220–7.

4

Women and schizophrenia: clinical aspects

Mary V. Seeman and Paul Fitzgerald

Schizophrenia is a disorder or group of disorders that presents in a heterogeneous manner. The symptomatic expression varies dramatically among individuals. Patterns in disease expression are slowly being identified as knowledge of the disorder grows. One of the most important areas in which differences in the expression of schizophrenia have been identified is that between women and men. As will be described, women with schizophrenia differ from men in their pattern of premorbid functioning, in the triggers that lead to psychotic episodes, in the clinical manifestation of specific symptoms and, importantly, in numerous dimensions of outcome.

These differences are multidetermined. Partially, this probably reflects brain sexual dimorphism, both structural and functional, evolved through millennia of genetic variation and selective pressures (see Chapter 2). Boys and girls display different behavioural repertoires from the earliest days following birth. In addition, they live in milieus that impose different role obligations on the two sexes, so that certain behaviours are habitually reinforced while others are extinguished by the responses and reactions of those around them. In most societies, males and females are not exposed to identical pressures or degrees of stress and, almost certainly, not to the same chronological timing of demands and expectations. None of this is specific to schizophrenia or to psychosis. None the less, these issues are likely to influence the way in which schizophrenia is manifest, as well as the responses of family and society to the patient with schizophrenia.

Premorbid competence and functioning

A number of studies have been carried out over the last 30 years that have looked at the premorbid functioning of patients with schizophrenia. The majority of these studies show premorbid functioning to be superior in young women relative to young men (Lewine, 1981; Aylward et al., 1984; Mueser et al., 1990a). This superiority is found in domains of social functioning, cognitive functioning, school and work achievement. Not all studies concur, however (Foerster et al., 1991), and there is disagreement as to proposed mechanisms that underlie these differences. Superior premorbid competence in women may reflect a faster pace of brain development and a later onset of illness. A later onset of illness means that women are able to achieve a higher level of social functioning prior to the development of their illness and to the social stagnation that this may bring (Hafner et al., 1995).

There is also evidence that neurodevelopmental factors play a role. Early onset, which is more common in males, may be particularly associated with a familial pattern of illness (Pulver et al., 1990; McGlashan & Fenton, 1991; Sham et al., 1994; see also Chapter 3). Such a pattern may be inherently more severe and also more likely to express itself early in life. Gender differences in the age of onset are not observed, however, in familial schizophrenia (Albus & Maier, 1995; DeLisi et al., 1994).

Research has indicated that males with schizophrenia have higher rates of obstetric complications and that this may be associated with a subset of schizophrenia characterized by early-onset and negative symptoms (Kirov et al., 1996). One recent study found that women with an early age of onset are likely to have experienced obstetric complications and to have very poor outcome (Gureje & Bamidele, 1998). It has also been proposed that a greater degree of lateralization of brain functions in males (McGlone, 1980) leaves them more vulnerable to the effects of a neurodevelopmental insult as there is less capacity for the brain to compensate by the use of the non-affected hemisphere (see Chapter 2).

Screening and illness detection

Schizophrenia starts later in women than in men (see Chapter 3). Trying systematically to determine when the symptoms of schizophrenia began (by detailed patient and family interview), investigators have shown that young women are generally symptomatic for somewhat longer before first diagnosis than are young men (Sartorius et al., 1978). This has significant implications for the prognosis of women with schizophrenia. In recent years evidence has increasingly emerged that delays in the commencement of antipsychotic drug treatment are associated with poorer outcomes in a number of domains. These include the length of time until illness remission, duration of remission and the degree of symptom response (Crow et al., 1986; Rabiner et al., 1986; Moscarelli et al., 1991; Loebel et al., 1992).

There are systematic and clinical impediments to the detection of early schizophrenia in women (Table 4.1). High school, military training, college and university are good screening grounds for early illness, and men usually develop schizophrenia at ages when they are likely to remain exposed to these institutions. Women, however, frequently do not become ill until they are out of the school setting, hidden away in the bosom of families, protected from would-be screeners. They may be relatively more sheltered by families for many reasons and this extra sheltering has often been thought of as conferring an advantage on women – a bulwark against the stressors that aggravate schizophrenic illness. Their relatively favourable early course has been pointed to as proof that extra sheltering pays off. This may prove, however, to be a double-edged sword as the duration of untreated symptoms may ultimately result in poorer outcomes. At this stage of our knowledge, the weight of the evidence is that early treatment – even when it involves the inevitable labelling and stigmatization – is, on balance, best for overall prognosis. The implication for women is that, if they came to medical attention earlier than they do, their outlook would not only remain better than men's, it would be incrementally better.

What is true of early-adult-onset schizophrenia is even more relevant to later-onset schizophrenia. After age 35, new cases of schizophrenia coming to medical attention are generally women (Castle et al., 1993). This group includes both women who have remained psychotic but hidden for a long period of time and women who have developed their psychosis at a later age. The onset of illness in this age group is not expected and the diagnosis can easily be missed because clinicians associate schizophrenia with adolescent onset. Furthermore, women with late-appearing schizophrenia may be quite accomplished, with their social skills intact, which is a deterrent to the

Table 4.1. Factors contributing to difficulties in early diagnosis in female patients

Prominence of affective symptoms
Relative lack of classical positive symptoms
Late age of onset
Infrequently exposed to routine screening (e.g. military settings)
Sheltering by protective family networks
Lack of clinical appreciation of atypical presentations

diagnosis of schizophrenia. Clinicians also associate schizophrenia with thought disorder and with negative symptoms which may be absent in late-appearing schizophrenia. Additionally, as detailed below, affective symptoms may be quite prominent. These difficulties with detection often mean that women may not be referred to specialized services and treatment may not be adequate. It is common, for instance, for women to be treated with antidepressant medications for a significant period of time before their psychotic disorder is recognized.

In the opinion of the present authors, the clinical lesson is that late-appearing psychotic symptoms in women may well mark the beginning of schizophrenia and should be treated promptly. The precise delineation between schizophrenia and affective psychosis is often less important than early recognition and treatment. Whether the illness is best conceptualized as affective psychosis with psychotic features or schizoaffective disorder is usually not clinically relevant. What is important is that antipsychotic drugs should be prescribed at effective doses and that psychotic features should not be allowed to persist.

Clinical features

Psychopathology and disease expression

The evolution and change in diagnostic criteria used to define this disorder have complicated the study of sex differences in the symptom patterns of patients with schizophrenia (see Chapter 3). It is generally accepted that women with psychotic disorders exhibit a broader range of symptoms than men, and that they often poorly fit the traditional view of the young patient with first-rank psychotic symptoms, negative symptoms and marked func-

Table 4.2. Sex differences in the expression of psychopathology in schizophrenia: characteristics reportedly more common in females

---

Superior premorbid functioning
Better preservation of social skills
Fewer negative symptoms (found in all ages)
Qualitative differences in the pattern of delusional ideation
Briefer and fewer hospitalizations

---

tional decline. The breadth of the criteria used to define schizophrenia will by necessity limit or include patients whose symptoms are atypical. It has been shown that the narrower the diagnostic criteria used, the more women are excluded from a diagnosis of schizophrenia (Lewine et al., 1984; Castle et al., 1993). The women thus excluded receive other diagnoses, presumably because of a prominent affective component to their presentation or because of the relative speed with which they recover from the index episode of psychosis.

Regardless of the age of onset, schizophrenia in women presents somewhat differently from that in men (Table 4.2). As has been discussed, there are differences in premorbid functioning but also in the pattern of clinical symptoms. Both clinical and epidemiological studies have shown that female patients have briefer and fewer hospitalizations and, overall, may have a less severe course of illness (Sartorius et al., 1978; Lewine, 1981; Lewine et al., 1984; Goldstein, 1988). When differences in diagnostic criteria are controlled for, female patients have also been found to have more mood features, fewer negative symptoms and better preserved social skills (Goldstein & Link, 1988; Childers & Harding, 1990; Shtasel et al., 1992).

There are also differences in the pattern of psychotic symptoms experienced by men and women (Allan & Hafner, 1989). Delusional themes in women may be less bizarre than in men, with more somatic preoccupation, erotomanic delusions, spiritual preoccupation, concern with interpersonal wrongs and relatively less worry about political espionage. Women have fewer homosexual persecutory delusions than do men, and fewer grandiose delusions involving personal power or status. They are more likely than men to experience delusions of pregnancy and of jealousy. For these reasons, women's delusions may be easier for clinicians to empathize with and fail to recognize as psychotic. The behaviour of women may also be more sedate (Kay et al., 1988; Sanguinetti et al., 1996) and less likely to attract attention. This may contribute to the previously discussed under-diagnosis and delay in treatment access.

Concurrent substance abuse

Comorbid substance abuse in schizophrenia is common (Reiger et al., 1990) and is associated with poorer outcome in terms of hospitalizations (Safer, 1987; Haywood et al., 1995), poorer treatment compliance and possibly illness relapse (Ayuso-Gutierrez & del Rio Vega, 1997). Rates and the patterns of substance abuse differ between the sexes. A greater propor-tion of men abuse drugs (Reiger et al., 1990; Ayuso-Gutierrez & del Rio Vega, 1997; De Quardo et al., 1994), including alcohol, cannabis and opiates, although one study has reported higher rates of stimulant abuse in women (Mueser et al., 1990b). In general, greater rates of male substance abuse in schizophrenia reflect the analogous situation in non-schizophrenic populations. In the general population, women drink less alcohol than men, begin drinking later but progress more quickly from the onset of drinking through later stages of alcoholism.

There is conflicting evidence as to the severity of substance abuse in female as compared to male patients with schizophrenia. As in the general population, female patients use lesser amounts of substances than do men (Test et al., 1989), although the severity of their substance abuse disorder may not differ (Brunette & Drake, 1997). Women with concurrent sub-stance use and psychotic disorders also appear more often to have more social contacts and be living with a partner or children than male patients with schizophrenia (Test et al., 1989; Brunette & Drake, 1997)

More alcoholic patients with schizophrenia report comorbid depression. They are also more likely to experience hallucinations (auditory, visual, gustatory, olfactory and tactile). More stigma is attached to women drinkers and the social sequelae in women are felt in their family life rather than in other domains of living (Brunette & Drake, 1997).

Triggering role of life events

Although part of well-accepted clinical experience, it has been difficult to prove conclusively whether life events trigger schizophrenia episodes, either initially or at subsequent relapse. The difficulties of proof are inherent in the measurement of the subjective impact of events and in ascertaining the degree to which the psychotic prodrome itself changes the subjective perception of an event or, indeed, elicits or causes the event.

The general population literature has documented that men and women are exposed to roughly equal numbers of life events but that women are more affected by them. The current view is that women perceive as stressful many events that men do not even report on a standardized questionnaire, namely problems of family, friends and neighbours (Dohrenwend & Dohrenwend, 1984). Kessler and colleagues (1981) analysed four epidemiological surveys of sex differences in life events and came to the conclusion that women are indeed more vulnerable to environmental occurrences than men, but only more vulnerable to those undesirable events that occur to others in their social network. Women appear to be more involved than men in support networks and, while this is generally considered a protective factor, it can be distressing, especially when one's network is more emotionally demanding than it is soothing.

One study has reported that life events trigger relapse in schizophrenia in women but not in men (Al Khani et al., 1986). In a somewhat different approach, van Os et al. (1994) performed a longitudinal follow-up of 166 patients (36% female) with psychotic illnesses and found that life events as a precipitant to psychotic relapse were associated with a relatively less severe, good-outcome illness.

Outcome

Outcome in patients with schizophrenia is complex and multidimensional. The course of illness and response to treatment vary between male and female patients in numerous ways. Sex differences are ubiquitous in areas of outcome that have been systematically studied.

Treatment outcome

The assessment of clinical response to neuroleptic medication is complicated by a number of factors. For instance, women have been reported to show higher neuroleptic plasma levels than men do after receiving the same dose of equivalent drug (Pollock, 1997; Yonkers et al., 1992). Some specific findings do emerge from the literature, however. One of the most consistent is that, in general, improved treatment responses have been reported for women both in time to remission and in dose required to achieve remission, although this appears to be limited to younger (premenopausal) women (Seeman, 1983). Baldessarini and colleagues (1995), for example, reported a 20% higher neuroleptic dose for men than for women in a hospital record study of 299 patients.

Furthermore, Salokangas (1995), reviewing a total of 1097 DSM-III-R schizophrenia patients over a 3-year post-hospital period, found no consistent increase in daily doses prescribed to women after menopause compared to premenopause. Szymanski et al. (1996) found no differences in response between a total of 69 treatment-refractory men and women treated with clozapine. Of course, the methodology of all these studies differs. Prescribed dose represents a synthesis of clinical wisdom but probably often reflects clinicians' biases more than patient requirements. Patient response, on the other hand, is dependent on many factors: demographic variables, lean-to-fat body ratio, smoking habits, menstrual regularity vs. amenorrhoea in women, use of concomitant drugs, illness history, types of symptoms, measures used to characterize response, dose conversion tables used, depot drug variables, drug wash-out periods, blind or non-blind conditions. With all these limitations, there remains the strong suggestion that a significant proportion of menstruating women who required maintenance neuroleptic doses which are relatively lower than that of their male-age peers when they are young subsequently require higher doses than their male counterparts in order to stay relapse-free. This change occurs around the time of menopause and may be as true for affective psychosis as for schizophrenia.

There is also some evidence that the response to psychosocial interventions may vary. The response to inpatient family intervention in a well-designed randomized trial was shown to be superior in women than men with schizophrenia (Haas et al., 1990), but it has also been shown that illness duration may be an important confound when interpreting male/female responsiveness to family treatment (Glick et al., 1990). One study has also indicated that the response to skill training may be worse in women (Schaub et al., 1998).

Cognitive outcome

Gender differences in cognitive symptom outcome in schizophrenia have only recently been addressed. Results depend on the chronicity of the sample, medication use, severity of negative symptoms, intelligence quotient, schooling and history of obstetric complications. In particular, age of onset may be an important confound, as early onset appears to correlate with poorer cognitive performance (Hoff et al., 1996). Specifics of the test battery applied and selection of control subjects also influence the results, making direct comparison across studies difficult.

Whilst several studies have reported worse cognitive performance in male schizophrenia patients (Haas et al., 1991; Hoff et al., 1992), others have reported worse function in female patients (Perlick et al., 1992) and others still report no gender differences (Goldberg et al., 1995). It appears likely that differences will be function-specific and may vary with illness subtype.

A recent large study by Lewine and colleagues (1997) indicates that sex and age of onset may interact in determining cognitive outcome. This investigation found some intersex differences (e.g. male patients scoring better than female patients on certain memory items) but the more dramatic findings appeared when age-of-onset comparisons were made within sexes. Specifically, this showed a worse cognitive outcome for early onset males (onset before age 25) compared to late-onset males, and poorer outcome for late-onset females when compared to early-onset females. The poorer-outcome patients were also judged to have less lateralized brain function. The results of this study and previously reported work from the same group (Lewine et al., 1995) indicate that cognitive deficits in female patients may predominantly relate to right hemisphere dysfunction or impaired information flow across the corpus callosum.

Disability outcome

The severity of illness expression is less debilitating in women than in men during the first decade following onset, but it worsens in subsequent years and eventually approximates that of men (Jonsson & Nyman, 1991; Opjordsmoen, 1991). This is true not only with respect to hospitalization variables such as number and frequency of admissions and lengths of stay, but also with respect to mental status at follow-up, social adaptation and occupational status.

Social outcome

The outcome of patients with schizophrenia has been studied in the area of a number of social variables. Two commonly used indexes of social outcome have been marital and reproductive rates, both of which vary with time and geography. In part because men have an earlier onset of illness, their marital rates are almost always shown to be lower than those of women (Nimgaonkar et al., 1997), but one study suggests that those men who do marry may have more children than their female counterparts (Lane et al., 1995). This is surprising since women with schizophrenia, in contrast to men, retain many of their interpersonal interests after illness onset. As stated, they continue to date and to be sexually active (see also Chapter 6).

There are also differences in the way in which males and females experience crime. Although men are more likely to be victims of crime – street crime, for instance – women live with more fear of its occurrence (Heidensohn, 1991). One reason for the fear may be the high rate of domestic crime committed against women, especially psychiatrically ill women, which is underestimated in some surveys and which may lead to the various sequelae of fear, isolation, avoidance and dependence.

Women comprise approximately 4% of the prison population because they commit only about 15% of serious offences and few of these are sufficiently dangerous to require custodial care (Heidensohn, 1991). One Swedish study has indicated that females with psychotic disorders are charged with a violent offence 27 times more than females without disorder, whereas the increase for males with a major mental illness is four times above a substantially higher baseline (Hodgins, 1992). The ratio of schizophrenia in women inmates relative to non-incarcerated woman is high but it is probably not as high as the 7:1 ratio reported for males with schizophrenia (Hodgins & Cote, 1990).

The homeless population tends to be 80% male, with the proportion of serious mental illness being roughly equal in men and women. Incidentally (and importantly for psychiatric prevention), homeless women are four to five times more likely than men to have children. In a study of intensive case management serving homeless shelter residents with psychiatric disability (not necessarily schizophrenia), Goering et al. (1992) found that, at entry into the programme, women had higher levels of social skills, larger and more supportive social networks and better housing conditions, but that these differences disappeared after 9 months in the programme. The programme provided both sexes with a similar quality of living conditions. It was hypothesized that equalizing housing conditions obliterated the initial differences between the sexes in social skills and social networks. In other words, this study suggests that such female advantages as exist may be secondary to standard of living.

Old-age outcome

Aging and the progress of schizophrenia occur side by side, making it impossible to disentangle the effects of age from the progress of disease. A number of long-term studies have tried to address questions with regard to the long-term outcome of this disorder. One of the most important studies in the area was the Lausanne 37-year follow-up study (Ciompi, 1980). This indicated that a significant number of patients experienced considerably fewer severe positive symptoms in old age, although negative symptoms tended to persist. Total outcome was judged favourable in half the cases followed. Despite the positive indicators, around one-third of patients remained or became severely disabled in old age (Ciompi, 1980).

Favourable outcome in old age was correlated with good premorbid social adjustment and less disturbed premorbid personality but, interestingly, there was no correlation with gender (Ciompi, 1985). In other words, even though relatively good premorbid adjustment correlates with female sex, by the end of life, what starts out as an advantage for women no longer is. Thus, whilst good premorbid adjustment still correlates with good old-age outcome, somewhere along the line more women than men have lost the protective power of that initial favourable start.

A more recent study has supported a number of the findings previously reported (Gur et al., 1996). In this prospective study of patients in a number of age groups, persistent sex differences in symptoms were found across all age groups. Whilst the study found that positive symptoms were the same for both sexes and fell with age for both, negative symptoms increased with age. In females, negative symptoms remained less severe at all ages.

Mortality outcome

In the general US population, life expectancy of females at birth currently exceeds that of males by approximately 10%. This is identical in other countries and has persisted over several centuries. Mortality among patients with schizophrenia has been consistently shown to be higher than in the general population in numerous large studies (Allebeck, 1989). Death rates are higher for suicide and other types of unnatural death as well as natural deaths such as cardiovascular disease (Newman & Bland, 1991). For example, in a study of 9156 patients first admitted with schizophrenia (a total national sample in Denmark), Mortensen & Juel (1993) examined rates and causes of death, and found the mortality ratio (death rate compared to the Danish general population) to be 4.7 in men with schizophrenia and 2.3 in women. The gender difference reflected the usual male/female dimorphism in mortality rates but the age-specific standardized mortality ratio was higher in women, especially in the younger age groups. Suicide accounted for 50% of the deaths in men and 35% of deaths in women – 20 times higher for both sexes than in the general population. Suicide rates were higher in men in all age groups, but relative risk of suicide for women was higher than in men until age 60. The risk for both sexes was particularly increased in the first follow-up year. Other violent causes of death were also increased in both sexes. Fatal accidents were four times more frequent and men with schizophrenia were victims of homicide almost 10 times more frequently than would be expected. Death from all natural causes except cancer and cerebrovascular disease was increased over that of the general population.

A meta-analysis of mortality in schizophrenia (Brown, 1997) indicated that there were no gender differences in natural-cause mortality, but the rate of unnatural-cause mortality was significantly higher in males.

Conclusions

Women with schizophrenia present differently from men, at different ages, and with different symptom patterns. Because of these differences, schizophrenia in women is often misdiagnosed. The course of illness is also different than in men with respect to both short- and long-term outcomes. These differences imply somewhat different approaches to therapeutic management. Whereas schizophrenia in men impacts primarily on the person who is ill, schizophrenia in women additionally exerts profound effects on spouses and on children. This calls for comprehensive family approaches which minimize harm and enhance functioning.

REFERENCES

Albus, M. & Maier, W. (1995). Lack of gender differences in age of onset in familial schizophrenia. *Schizophr. Res.,* **18**, 51–7.

Al Khani, M., Bebbington, P., Watson J., et al. (1986). Life events and schizophrenia. A Saudi Arabian study. *Br. J. Psychiatry,* **148**, 12–22.

Allan, J. & Hafner, R. (1989). Sex differences in the phenomenology of schizophrenic disorder. *Can. J. Psychiatry,* **34**, 46–8.

Allebeck, P. (1989). Schizophrenia: a life shortening disease. *Schizophr. Bull.,* **15**, 81–9.

Aylward, E., Walker, E. & Bettes, B. (1984). Intelligence in schizophrenia: meta-analysis of the research. *Schizophr. Bull.,* **10**, 430–59.

Ayuso-Gutierrez, J. & del Rio Vega, J. (1997). Factors influencing relapse in the long-term course of schizophrenia. *Schizophr. Res.,* **28**, 199–206.

Baldessarini, R., Kando, J. & Centovieno, F. (1995). Hospital use of antipsychotic agents in 1989 and 1993: Stable dosing with decreased length of stay. *Am. J. Psychiatry,* **152**, 1038–44.

Brown, S. (1997). Excess mortality in schizophrenia. *Br. J. Psychiatry,* **171**, 502–8.

Brunette, M. & Drake, R. (1997). Gender differences in patients with schizophrenia and substance abuse. *Compr. Psychiatry,* **38**, 109–16.

Castle, D.J., Wessely, S. & Murray, R.M. (1993). Sex and schizophrenia: effects of diagnostic stringency, and associations with premorbid variables. *Br. J. Psychiatry,* **162**, 658–64

Childers, S. & Harding, C. (1990). Gender, premorbid social functioning and long term outcome in DSM III-schizophrenia. *Schizophr. Bull.,* **16**, 309–18

Ciompi, L. (1980). Catamnestic long-term study on the course of life and aging of schizophrenics. *Schizophr. Bull.,* **6**, 606–18.

Ciompi, L. (1985). Aging and schizophrenic psychosis. *Acta Psychiatr. Scand.,* **71** (suppl. 319), 93–105.

Crow, T., MacMillian, J., Johnson, A. et al. (1986). A randomised trial of prophylactic neuroleptic treatment. *Br J. Psychiatry,* **148**, 120–7.

DeLisi, L., Bass, N., Boccio, A. et al. (1994). Age of onset in familial schizophrenia. *Arch. Gen. Psychiatry,* **51**, 334–5.

De Quardo, J., Carpenter, C. & Tandon, R. (1994). Patterns of substance abuse in schizophrenia: nature and significance. *J. Psychiatr. Res.,* **28**, 267–75.

Dohrenwend B.S. & Dohrenwend, B.P. (1984). *Stressful Life Events: Their Nature and Effect.* New York: Wiley.

Foerster, A., Lewis, S., Owen, M. et al. (1991). Pre-morbid adjustment and personality in psychosis. Effects of sex and diagnosis. *Br. J. Psychiatry,* **158**, 171–6.

Glick, I., Spencer, J., Clarkin, J. et al. (1990). A randomised clinical trial of inpatient family intervention. IV. Follow up results for subjects with schizophrenia. *Schizophr. Res.,* **3**, 187–200.

Goering, P., Wasylenki, D., Onge, M. et al. (1992). Gender differences among clients of a case management program for the homeless. *Hosp. Commun. Psychiatry*, **43**, 160–5.

Goldberg, T., Gold, J., Torrey, E. et al. (1995). Lack of sex differences in the neuropsychological performance of patients With schizophrenia. *Am. J. Psychiatry*, **152**, 883–8.

Goldstein, J. (1988). Gender differences in the course of schizophrenia. *Am. J. Psychiatry*, **145**, 684–9.

Goldstein, J. & Link, B. (1988). Gender and the expression of schizophrenia. *J. Psychiatr. Res.*, **22**, 141–55.

Gur, R., Petty, R., Turetsky, B. et al. (1996). Schizophrenia throughout life: sex differences in severity and profile of symptoms. *Schizophr. Res.*, **21**, 1–12.

Gureje, O. & Bamidele, R. (1998). Gender and schizophrenia: association of age at onset with antecedent, clinical and outcome features. *Aust. N.Z. J. Psychiatry*, **32**, 415–23.

Haas, G., Glick, I., Clarkin, J. et al. (1990). Gender and schizophrenia outcome: a clinical trial of inpatient family intervention. *Schizophr. Bull.*, **16**, 277–92.

Haas, G., Sweeney, J., Hien, D. et al. (1991). Gender differences in schizophrenia. *Schizophr. Res.*, **4**, 277.

Hafner, H., Nowotny, B., Loffler, W. et al. (1995). When and how does schizophrenia produce social deficits? *Eur. Arch. Psychiatry Clin. Neurosci.*, **246**, 17–28.

Haywood, T., Kravitz, H., Grossman, L. et al. (1995). Predicting the 'revolving door' phenomena among patients with schizophrenic, schizoaffective and affective disorders. *Am. J. Psychiatry*, **152**, 856–61.

Heidensohn, F. (1991). Women as perpetrators and victims of crime. *Br. J. Psychiatry*, **158** (Suppl. 10), 50–4.

Hodgins, S. (1992). Mental disorder, intellectual deficiency, and crime: evidence from a birth cohort. Gen. Psychiatry, **49**, 476–83.

Hodgins, S. & Cote, G. (1990). Prevalence of mental disorders among penitentiary inmates in Quebec. *Can. Mental Health*, March, 1–4.

Hoff, A., Riordan, H. & DeLisi, L. (1992). Influence of gender on neuropsychological testing and MRI measures of schizophrenic inpatients. *Schizophr. Bull.*, **82**, 257–72.

Hoff, A., Harris, D., Faustman, W. et al. (1996). A neuropsychological study of early onset schizophrenia. *Schizophr. Res.*, **20**, 21–8.

Jonsson, H. & Nyman, A. (1991). Predicting long-term outcome in schizophrenia. *Acta Psychiatr. Scand.*, **83**, 342–6.

Kay, S., Wolkenfeld, F. & Murrill, L. (1988). Profiles of aggression among psychiatric patients: II Covariates and predictors. *J. Nerv. Ment. Dis.*, **176**, 547–57.

Kessler, R., Brown, R. & Broman, C. (1981). Sex differences in psychiatric help-seeking: Evidence from four large scale sureys. *J. Health Soc. Behav.*, **22**, 49–64.

Kirov, G., Jones, P., Rifkin, L. et al. (1996). Do obstetric complications cause the earlier age at onset in male than female schizophrenics? *Schizophr. Res.*, **20**, 117–24.

Lane, A., Byrne, M., Mulvaney, F. et al. (1995). Reproductive behavior in schizophrenia relative to other mental disorders: evidence for increased fertility in men despite a decreased marital rate. *Acta Psychiatr. Scand.*, **91**, 222–8.

Lewine, R. (1981). Sex differences in schizophrenia: timing of subtypes? *Psychol. Bull.*, **90**, 423–44.

Lewine, R., Burbach, D. & Meltzer, H. (1984). Effect of diagnostic criteria on the ratio of male to female schizophrenic patients. *Am. J. Psychiatry*, **141**, 84–7.

Lewine, R., Walker, E., Shurett, R. et al. (1995). Sex differences in neuropsychological functioning among schizophrenic patients. *Am. J. Psychiatry*, **153**, 1178–84.

Lewine, R., Haden, C., Caudle, J. et al. (1997). Sex-onset effects on neuropsychological function in schizophrenia. *Schizophr. Bull.*, **23**, 51–61.

Loebel, A., Lieberman, J., Alvir, J. et al. (1992). Duration of psychosis and outcome in first-episode schizophrenia. *Am. J. Psychiatry*, **149**, 1183–8.

McGlashan, T. & Fenton, W. (1991). Classical subtypes for schizophrenia: literature review for DSM-IV. *Schizophr. Bull.*, **17**, 609–23.

McGlone, J. (1980). Sex differences in human brain asymmetry: a critical survey. *Behav. Brain Sci.*, **3**, 215–63.

Meuser, K., Bellack, A., Morrison, R. et al. (1990a). Social competence in schizophrenia: Premorbid adjustment, social skill, and domains of functioning. *J. Psychiatr. Res.*, **24**, 51–63.

Meuser, K., Yarnold, P., Levinson, D. et al. (1990b). Prevalence of substance abuse in schizophrenia: demographics and clinical correlates. *Schizophr. Bull.*, **16**, 31–56.

Mortensen, P. & Juel, K. (1993). Mortality and causes of death in first admitted schizophrenic patients. *Br. J. Psychiatry*, **163**, 183–9.

Moscarelli, M., Capri, S. & Neri, L. (1991). Cost evaluation of chronic schizophrenic patients during the first 3 years after the first contact. *Schizophr. Bull.*, **17**, 421–6.

Newman, S. & Bland, R. (1991). Mortality in a cohort of patients with schizophrenia: A record linkage study. *Can. J. Psychiatry*, **36**, 239–45.

Nimgaonkar, V., Ward, S., Agarde, H. et al. (1997). Fertility in schizophrenia: results from a contemporary US cohort. *Acta Psychiatr. Scand.*, **95**, 364–9.

Opjordsmoen, S. (1991). Long-term clinical outcome of schizophrenia with special reference to gender differences. *Acta Psychiatr. Scand.*, **83**, 307–13.

Perlick, D., Mattis, S., Stastny, P. et al. (1992). Gender differences in cognition in schizophrenia. *Schizophr. Res.*, **8**, 69–73.

Pollock, B. (1997). Gender differences in psychotropic drug metabolism. *Psychopharmacol. Bull.*, **241**, 235–41.

Pulver, A., Brown, C., Wolyniec, P. et al. (1990). Schizophrenia: age at onset , gender and familial risk. *Acta Psychiatr. Scand.*, **82**, 344–51.

Rabiner, C., Wegner, J. & Kane, J. (1986). Outcome of first-episode psychosis: 1. Relapse rates after 1 year. *Am. J. Psychiatry*, **143**, 1155–8.

Rieger, D., Farmer, M., Rae, D. et al. (1990). Comorbidity of mental disorders with alcohol and drug abuse: results from the Epidemiologic Catchment Area (ECA) study. *JAMA*, **264**, 2511–18.

Safer, D. (1987). Substance use by young adult chronic patients. *Hosp. Commun. Psychiatry*, **38**, 511–14.

Salokangas, R. (1995). Gender and the use of neuroleptics in schizophrenia. Further testing of the estrogen hypothesis. *Schizophr. Res.*, **16**, 7–16.

Sanguinetti, V., Samuel, S., Schwartz, S. et al. (1996). Gender differences among civilly committed schizophrenia subjects. *Schizophr. Bull.*, **22**, 653–8.

Sartorius, N., Jablensky, A. & Shapiro, R. (1978). Cross-cultural differences in the short-term prognosis of schizophrenia psychosis. *Schizophr. Bull.*, **4**, 102–13.

Schaub, A., Behrendt, B., Brenner, H. et al. (1998). Training schizophrenic patients to manage their symptoms: predictors of treatment response to the German version of the Symptom Management Module. *Schizophr. Res.*, **31**, 121–30.

Seeman, M.V. (1983). Interaction of sex, age and neuroleptic dose. *Compr. Psychiatry*, **24**, 125–8.

Sham, P., Jones, P., Russell A. et al. (1994). Age at onset, sex, and familial psychiatric morbidity in schizophrenia: Camberwell collaborative psychosis study. *Br. J. Psychiatry*, **165**, 466–73.

Shtasel, D., Gur, R., Gallacher, F. et al. (1992). Gender differences in the clinical expression of schizophrenia. *Schizophr. Res.*, **7**, 225–31.

Szymanski, S., Lieberman, J., Pollack, S. et al. (1996). Gender differences in neuroleptic nonresponsive clozapine-treated schizophrenics. *Biol. Psychiatry*, **39**, 249–54.

Test, M., Yallisch, L. & Ripp, K. (1989). Substance use in the young adults with schizophrenic disorders. *Schizophr. Bull.*, **15**, 465–76.

van Os, J., Fahy, T., Bebbington, P. et al. (1994). The influence of life events on the subsequent course of psychotic illness: a follow-up of the Camberwell Collaborative Psychosis Study. *Psychol. Med.*, **24**, 503–513

Yonkers, K., Kando, J. C., Cole, J. et al. (1992). Gender differences in pharmacokinetics and pharmacodynamics of psychotropic medication. *Am. J. Psychiatry*, **149**, 587–95.

5

Hormones and psychosis

Jayashri Kulkarni and George Fink

In 1892, Emil Kraepelin postulated links between hormones and dementia praecox and undertook endocrine reviews of his patients. Other early researchers such as Hoskins (1929) studied endocrine changes in schizophrenia in postmortem studies. During this period, the discovery of insulin stimulated further interest in the interaction of behaviour and metabolism. Hoskin's work ultimately discounted the efficacy of treating schizophrenia by insulin-induced hypoglycaemia and provided an important early focus on endocrine research in schizophrenia.

Between 1940 and 1970, there was considerable interest in the psychoendocrine characterization of schizophrenia. The mimicking of psychotic symptoms by the administration of high doses of steroid hormones (Mason, 1975) and the demonstration of elevated levels of the steroid metabolic 17–hydroxycorticosteroid in acutely ill people with schizophrenia (Sachar et al., 1963) were two important early neuroendocrine studies in schizophrenia. Brambilla & Penati (1978) reviewed the evidence for hypo- and hyperfunction of the adrenal, pituitary and thyroid glands, and of the gonads, in patients with schizophrenia. Endocrinopathies were only rarely present, suggesting that endocrine abnormalities in these patients were due to the disease process of schizophrenia rather than being causally related.

With increasing clarity of the role of neurotransmitters in the regulation of pituitary hormone release via hypothalamic hormones, neuroendocrine studies in schizophrenia conducted in the early 1980s aimed to use the pituitary gland as the window on the brain, using probes that modified the secretion of anterior pituitary hormones to detect abnormalities in tubero-infundibular–pituitary function, reflecting similar abnormalities in the mesolimbic system. In a review of this area, Lieberman & Koreen (1993) concluded that the hypothalamic–pituitary–thyroid axis in general has not been shown to manifest disturbances specific to schizophrenia. Nevertheless, studies of growth hormone have tended to show a response to a wide variety of pharmacological probes (e.g. apomorphine, tryptophan, fenfluramine, baclofen, clonidine, methylphenidate and bromocriptine), suggestive of enhanced noradrenergic activity in patients with schizophrenia compared with controls. Studies of prolactin, on the other hand, have tended to show a blunted response in schizophrenia to probes such as haloperidol (Keks et al., 1987). A blunted cortisol response to hypoglycaemic stress has also been demonstrated (Lerer et al., 1988; Kathol et al., 1992).

A clear omission from the neuroendocrine studies described to date is females. Researchers have often excluded women because of a putative inability to control for the variable of fluctuating monthly hormonal cycles.

Puerperal psychosis

Historically, mental-state changes have been linked with biological events related to the female reproductive system. 'Puerperal insanity' has been described as a clearly recognizable disorder from very early times. A study of postpartum psychosis in nineteenth- compared with twentieth-century women suggested that little has changed in the clinical presentation (Anis-Ur-Rehman et al., 1990), and that puerperal psychosis manifests as a mixed picture of affective and psychotic symptoms. Many clinicians would agree that puerperal psychosis poses unique diagnostic and therapeutic challenges worthy of a separate category (Kane, 1985); yet current classification systems (DSM-IV) include this group of female psychotic disorders with all other psychoses.

There are relatively few neuroendocrine studies involving women suffering from puerperal psychosis. Kumar et al. (1983) detailed the difficulties in recruiting neuroleptic-free psychotic postpartum women for neuroendocrine studies, but underlined the need to use current biomedical technology to allow testing of neuroendocrine hypotheses about the aetiology of postpartum psychosis. George & Sandler (1988) reviewed biological theories of postpartum psychosis and related psychiatric symptoms to 'hormonal shock', which is the abrupt reduction after parturition of massive levels of many hormones that had gradually increased during pregnancy.

Studies by Nott et al. (1976) and Kuevi et al. (1983), investigating the relationship between the fall in estradiol levels and puerperal psychosis, were performed on small samples and produced conflicting results. Wieck et al. (1991), measuring growth hormone response to apomorphine challenge in 8 postpartum women, revealed an increased sensitivity of hypothalamic dopamine. The role of prolactin in puerperal psychoses remains unclear, but some researchers (George et al., 1980; Kuevi et al., 1983) have reported a correlation between plasma prolactin and puerperal disorders. However, these studies reported wide individual variations in plasma prolactin concentrations due to suckling. The peptide hormone beta-endorphin has been shown to be significantly decreased in women with severe postpartum depression (George & Wilson, 1982; Newham et al., 1984) but has not been measured in women with psychosis. Clearly, there is a need for further neuroendocrine work in the area of puerperal psychosis, with a major challenge being the standardization of hormonal fluctuations in control subjects and patients to enable comparison.

The menstrual cycle and psychosis

Hippocrates (460–377 BC) and his followers subscribed to the view that a woman was dominated by her uterus and the menstrual cycle, and that the pathological shifting of the uterus was the cause of mental disorders (Rosen, 1968). The popular view of the late Middle Ages was that menstruation itself caused madness, and menstruating women spread madness and were to be avoided (Scot, 1534). Even in the nineteenth century, menstruation and its abnormalities were assumed to be one of the important causes of psychosis; the diagnosis 'menstruation psychose' was a popular one in Kraepelin's time.

Biological research in schizophrenia, particularly neurochemical and neuroendocrinological studies, often excludes women or ignores menstrual-cycle effects. Reasons include a lack of consistency in the definition of menstrual phases. In order to include women in biological schizophrenia research studies, their menstrual-cycle phase needs to be reliably determined and biologically confirmed. A Menstrual Distress Questionnaire was developed by Moos in 1968, but the object of this questionnaire was mainly to record symptoms of premenstrual syndrome (PMS). The Menstrual Cycle Interview (Kulkarni et al., 1996b) is an attempt to ascertain reliable cycle-phase estimation from women with schizophrenia, and it is hoped that future biological schizophrenia research will include women as participants and also study cycle phase as an important potential confounding factor.

Literature supporting a close association between menstrual-cycle phase and psychosis exacerbation or onset is mainly found in the form of case reports and anecdotal clinical reports. Endo and colleagues (1978) have perhaps provided the most detailed study of psychosis recurring with the menstrual cycle. These researchers followed the progress of 7 patients who had diagnosed psychotic illness over a 10-year period. In all 7 subjects, psychotic episodes occurred regularly, with exacerbation of symptoms beginning 5–10 days premenstrually and resolving after menstruation ceased in all cases. These women would have met criteria for 'periodic psychosis', which has been widely described (Lingjaerde & Bredland, 1954; Dalton, 1959; Hatotani et al., 1959; Felthous et al., 1980; Berlin et al., 1982; Vogel et al., 1992).

Dalton (1959) demonstrated that female patients with known psychiatric illness were more likely to be admitted to hospital with an exacerbation of illness in the premenstrual or menstrual phase. Other more recent studies (Abramowitz et al., 1982; Luggin et al., 1984; Hallonquist et al., 1993) detail an increase in symptom severity and hence hospital admissions in the premenstrual and menstruation phases in women with diagnosed schizophrenia. Vogel et al. (1992) found a significant excess of admissions in the paramenstruum for 65 women with schizophrenia, whilst Riecher-Rossler et al. (1994) studied 32 acutely psychotic women, and found a significant excess of admissions in the premenstrual and menstruation phases, with an inverse relationship between serum estradiol and severity of psychotic symptoms.

Menstrual-cycle abnormalities also include a diverse collection of physical and mental symptoms termed the premenstrual syndrome or PMS. Studies of PMS in women with psychotic disorders have been hampered by problems in standardizing methodology for data collection in staging the menstrual-cycle phase and in defining the range of symptoms. An early study (Torghele, 1957) reported increased PMS symptoms in psychotic women. Zola et al. (1979) did not confirm this, but did find that women with psychosis experienced an exacerbation of psychotic symptoms in the paramenstruum.

The estrogen protection hypothesis

Pioneering researchers in the area of sex differences in the onset, treatment and outcome of schizophrenia, such as Lewine (1988), Seeman & Lang (1990) and Hafner (1991), have proposed that in women estrogen may confer protection against the early onset of severe schizophrenia. Furthermore, these researchers have suggested that women are vulnerable to relapses of schizophrenia or their first episode of illness in the perimenopausal period, when estrogen production diminishes. As articulated by Hafner et al. (1998), the hypothesis also encompasses early estrogen effects on the developing brain, such that a structural effect of estrogen acting already during brain maturation causes the delay of first onset in females by raising the vulnerability threshold for schizophrenia. From puberty, this putative structural effect is reinforced by a functional effect, as detailed above. Fading estrogen secretion around menopause causes women predisposed for schizophrenia, but who until then have been protected by estrogens, to fall ill with late-onset schizophrenia.

Essentially, the estrogen protection hypothesis rests on three broad lines of work: epidemiological studies; biological or basic science studies using animal models; and clinical studies (Hafner et al., 1998).

Epidemiological studies

A sex difference in the age at first admission, with women being older than men, was noted by Kraepelin in 1909. The finding was largely ignored until the late 1980s, when Angermeyer & Kuhn (1988) confirmed the age difference at first admission in 50 out of 53 international studies (see also Chapter 3).

Using large population samples from the Danish and Mannheim (Germany) case registers, Hafner and colleagues (1990) confirmed significant gender differences in age at first admission (4–5 years), and in age at first onset of symptoms (3–4 years). A review of possible artefactual reasons for the gender differences in prevalence and incidence rates with respect to treatment-seeking, conducted by Hambrecht et al. (1992), concluded that the consistent finding of an earlier age of onset of schizophrenia in men compared with women has transnational stability. A second and also important gender difference is the significant increase in the incidence of first presentations of psychosis in women aged 45–49 years (Hafner et al., 1998). For a further discussion of these issues, the reader is referred to Chapter 3.

Animal models

Behrens and colleagues (1992) studied the effects of estradiol and testosterone on cataplexy induced by the dopamine antagonist haloperidol in neonatal and adult rats. Oral stereotypies, grooming and sitting behaviour induced by the dopamine agonist were also studied after administration of estradiol and testosterone. Estradiol was noted to reduce significantly the behavioural changes induced by both haloperidol and apomorphine, while testosterone did not. Behrens et al. (1992) concluded that these results suggest a down-regulation of dopamine neurotransmission by estradiol. This conclusion does not account for the positive effect that estradiol had on haloperidol-induced cataplexy, since up-regulation of dopamine neurotransmission would be required for behavioural improvement to occur.

The actions of estrogen on the dopamine system are complex, and effects of estrogen on dopaminergic neurotransmissions are believed to depend on the dose and length of administration. Studies have demonstrated that within 24 h of low-dose estradiol being administered to rats, there is a significant decrease in the ratio of high- to low-affinity agonist states of the striatal dopamine D_2 receptors (Gordon et al., 1980; Di Paolo et al., 1982; Joyce et al., 1982); this has been described as an acute hyposensitive state. On the other hand, administration of high doses of estrogen results in the development of striatal dopamine receptor hypersensitivity (Perry et al., 1981; Clopton & Gordon, 1986). This can be expressed behaviourally in rats as an increase in dopamine agonist-induced stereotypes, or biochemically as an increase in the density of $[^3H]$ spiroperidol-binding sites (Gordon et al., 1980; Gordon & Perry, 1983). Ferretti et al. (1992) found that estrogen administration had little effect on dopamine D_1 receptors, but that D_2 receptor density fell in response to low-dose estradiol. These workers also reported that administration of high-dose estradiol resulted in supersensitivity of D_1 receptors in male rats. Other studies have described an increase in the density of striatal dopamine receptors when estradiol was administered chronically (Hruska et al., 1980; Di Paolo et al., 1982).

More recently, Fink and colleagues (1998, 1999) have shown that estrogen induces a significant increase in $5\text{-}HT_{2A}$ receptors and the serotonin transporter (SERT) in regions of the rat forebrain that, in humans, are concerned with mental state, mood, cognition, memory, emotion and neuroendocrine control. The precise mechanism of the estrogen–serotonin interaction is not clear. However, the forebrain receives a dense innervation of serotonergic projections from the midbrain raphe neurones, and the $5\text{-}HT_{2A}$ receptors are present at high concentrations in most areas of forebrain and especially the anterior and frontal cingulate cortex – regions of the forebrain concerned with cognition and emotion. The highest density of these receptors is in laminae IV and VA of these regions of the cortex, where the receptors are located on the apical dendrites of the pyramidal neurones and on glutamatergic interneurones.

The net effect of 5-HT stimulation of the $5\text{-}HT_{2A}$ receptors in frontal and cingulate cortex would probably be to increase the rate of firing of the pyramidal neurones, although this might be offset by inhibitory effects mediated by $5\text{-}HT_1$ receptors. Since the functional density of 5-HT receptors will be influenced by the concentrations of 5-HT to which they are exposed, the density and degree of activity of serotonin transporters (SERT) may also have a bearing on $5\text{-}HT_{2A}$ receptor activity. However, the estrogen-induced increase in the density of SERT sites occurs in areas of the forebrain (amygdala, lateral septum and venteromedial nucleus of the hypothalamus) in which estrogen has no apparent effect on the density of the $5\text{-}HT_{2A}$ receptors.

The action of estrogen on $5\text{-}HT_{2A}$ receptors and the SERT could be mediated by both genomic and non-genomic mechanisms. Fink et al. (1998) reported that estrogen induced a two- to threefold increase in the amount of $5HT_{2A}$ receptor messenger RNA in the dorsal raphe nucleus, suggesting that exposure to estrogen stimulated $5HT_{2A}$ receptor gene transcription. This is in contrast to the finding of an estrogen-induced rise in $5HT_{2A}$ receptor density without a concordant rise in $5HT_{2A}$ receptor messenger RNA in cortical neurones. This is analogous to the action of estradiol on D_2 receptor-expressing neurons in the striatum, where there are few estradiol receptors. The action of estradiol in the striatum may be mediated by membrane rather than classical cytoplasmic receptors. Mosselman et al. (1996) cloned a second estrogen receptor and termed it estrogen receptor-beta (as distinct from estrogen receptor-alpha). Shughrue et al. (1997), Fink et al. (1998) and Sumner et al. (1999) have provided data that suggest that any genomic action of estrogen on the $5HT_{2A}$ receptor and SERT genes may be mediated by the estrogen receptor-beta.

Estrogen, by way of its actions on the $5\text{-}HT_{2A}$ receptor, the SERT and the D_2 receptor, may protect against depressive and psychotic symptoms. This apparent psychoprotective effect of estrogen may have a major biological purpose in that teleologically, the actions of estrogen may be related to its role as the major endocrine coordinator of events that lead to fertility and therefore reproduction. Estrogen triggers the ovulatory luteinizing hormone-releasing hormone/luteinizing hormone surge which influences mating behaviour in nonhuman primates. In order for mating to occur, mood and mental state must be right in both humans and other animals. Hence estrogen triggers and coordinates several biological events which are necessary for procreation.

The significance of these findings for schizophrenia lies in the fact that the $5HT_{2A}$ receptor is the target for the atypical antipsychotics, such as olanzapine and clozapine, which are especially effective in the treatment of the negative symptoms of the illness (Fink, 1995). Thus, the effect of estrogen on $5\text{-}HT_{2A}$ receptors could be part of the explanation for the findings encompassed in the estrogen protection hypothesis. There is no conflict between the possible involvement of serotonin and the dopamine hypothesis of schizophrenia, since estrogen increased density of both the dopamine D_2, and the $5HT_{2A}$ receptor, such that the two mechanisms could operate in parallel (Fink, 1995; Fink et al., 1998).

Clinical studies

A full discussion of the clinical aspects of women with schizophrenia is provided in Chapter 4. Here we mention only those studies of women with schizophrenia which have taken account of menstrual phase and/or gonadal hormone level.

Clinically, there have been case reports of psychotic symptoms occurring cyclically in women with schizophrenia during the late luteal phase when estrogen levels are at their lowest (Dalton, 1959; Endo et al., 1978). Riecher-Rossler and colleagues (1992) tested the hypothesis that the symptomatology of schizophrenia varied with the menstrual cycle phase in 32 acutely admitted women who gave a history of regular cycles. They found a significant excess of admissions during the premenstrual (i.e. low-estrogen phase) compared with the high-estrogen phase. This study also found a significant inverse relationship between estradiol levels and severity of psychotic symptoms. Furthermore, all 32 patients had markedly low estradiol levels throughout the cycle.

Seeman (1983) reported that neuroleptic dose requirements in psychotic women rise as they approach menopause and described premenopausal women as 'already neuroleptized by their antidopaminergic oestrogens'. Seeman attributed an increased vulnerability to psychosis in the postmenopause period to the fall in circulating estrogen levels.

The psychiatric literature contains case reports of women suffering from psychotic symptoms perimenstrually (Lingjaerde & Bredland, 1954; Berlin et al., 1982). There are also reports of improvement in psychotic symptoms with the addition of a combined estrogen–progesterone oral contraceptive (Felthous et al., 1980; Dennerstein et al., 1983). In an 8-week open clinical trial, Kulkarni and colleagues (1996a) found that 11 acutely psychotic women who received 0.02 mg oral estradiol as an adjunct to antipsychotic drug treatment made a more rapid improvement in psychotic symptoms than a control group who received antipsychotic drug treatments alone. In a recent 4-week double-blind placebo-controlled study, Kulkarni and colleagues (1996b) found that 13 premenopausal women with psychosis who received 100 µg estradiol skin patches plus antipsychotic medication had significantly lower total Positive and Negative Syndrome Scale (PANSS: Kay et al., 1987) and Brief Psychiatric Rating Scale (BPRS: Overall & Gorham, 1962) scores than did 13 psychotic women who received placebo patches plus antipsychotic medication. The greater improvement in psychotic symptoms in the estrogen-adjunct group was in all symptom subscale of the PANSS.

Clearly, the estrogen protection hypothesis requires further rigorous testing, and estrogen alone cannot account for the extent of gender differences in schizophrenia, as articulated in Chapter 4. However, the hypothesis provides some rationale for the consideration of the role of estrogen in both the aetiogenesis of gender differences in schizophrenia and in the development of specific treatments for women with schizophrenia.

Hormonal treatments for women with schizophrenia

The treatment aspects of schizophrenia in women are presented in Chapter 8. Here we provide a brief review of hormonal treatments. It should be stressed that the area of hormone treatments for women with schizophrenia is a speculative one, based on theory and still awaiting conclusive clinical trials. However, there are some safe treatment options that clinicians can already utilize.

Adjunctive hormone replacement therapy for postmenopausal women with schizophrenia

Many clinicians will have noted a deterioration in mental state in women with existing schizophrenia as they approach menopause. While there are a number of contributing factors, many of which are psychosocial in nature, the biological advent of declining circulating estrogen and/or the preceding elevation in pituitary gonadotrophin levels (luteinizing hormone, follicle-stimulating hormone) may be a major contributing factor.

Hormone replacement therapy (HRT) is currently an option for assisting women who experience troubling symptoms such as hot flushes, or to aid in preventing osteoporosis and cardiovascular morbidity. More recently, HRT has been noted to have positive effects on cognition and mood in menopausal women. Thus, menopausal women with schizophrenia may benefit from HRT in terms of their mental state and physical health. A further reason to consider HRT in menopausal women with schizophrenia is to counter the unwanted hyperprolactinaemia effects that may have accompanied a lifetime of treatment with older antipsychotic medication. These issues are detailed further in Chapter 8.

Adjunctive estrogen treatment in premenopausal women with schizophrenia

The clinical trials conducted to date and detailed in this chapter suggest that estrogen may be a useful addition to antipsychotic medication in terms of down-regulating dopaminergic transmission and by its action on serotonin metabolism. However, the appropriate dose, longer-term effects and concomitant progesterone administration are yet to be determined. None the less, the adjunctive use of a combined estrogen–progesterone preparation may be a useful treatment adjunct in those women with demonstrated monthly cyclical relapse in illness. Modified HRT could also be used to deliver more physiological doses of estrogen across each menstrual cycle.

Selective estrogen receptor modulators

A potentially useful adjunct in the future is the selective estrogen receptor modulators (SERMs), which are estrogen compounds that influence central nervous system neurotransmitter systems without affecting breast or uterine tissue. The major potential risks in using estrogen as a longer-term treatment in women are the potentially harmful effects of estrogen on breast and uterine tissue. For this reason SERMs may be a better option, especially in premenopausal women. An early SERM is raloxifene, whose action is mediated by binding to estrogen receptors and thereby regulating gene expression. Raloxifene is inferred to impact on dopamine and serotonin pathways in a similar fashion to conjugated estrogens (Nickelsen et al., 1999). Since SERMs have only recently been developed, there are few clinical studies on their action and no information is yet available on their effect on psychotic symptoms.

A possible role for progesterone in women with schizophrenia?

Progesterone and related steroids are thought to exert a sedative/anaesthetic effect (Hackmann et al., 1973; Cone et al., 1981). Estrogen induces brain progesterone receptors (McEwen et al., 1981; Alves et al., 1998), hence the action of estrogen could be mediated, in part, by progesterone. Estrogen may potentiate the sedative action of progesterone by stimulating an increase in progesterone receptors during the luteal phase of the menstrual cycle and during pregnancy. The precipitous drop in plasma progesterone concentrations at the end of the luteal phase may account for anxiety symptoms in the premenstrual phase (Fink et al., 1998).

It has been a relatively common practice to use a long-acting intramuscular progesterone-only compound as a contraceptive in women with schizophrenia. The addition of exogenous progesterone without estrogen may inhibit the production of estrogen by the ovaries, thereby potentially being counterproductive in the central nervous system in terms of dopamine and serotonin metabolism. Clinical studies investigating this speculation have not been conducted, although the use of depot progesterone as a contraception has declined. The role of progesterone-only preparations as treatment in postpartum depression has been advocated by Dalton (1980) and Solthau & Taylor (1982), but its therapeutic success in the puerperium has not been substantiated by controlled clinical trials.

Conclusions

The subjective observations by women with schizophrenia that there may be a correlation between changes in their menstrual cycle and the onset or subsequent relapse of psychotic symptoms appears to have some basis in epidemiological, biological and psychopathological schizophrenia studies. However, hormonal research in women with schizophrenia is still in its infancy and more controlled clinical trials are required before clear aetiologies can be determined, or definitive treatment options defined.

REFERENCES

Abramowitz, E.S., Baker, A.H. & Fleischer, S.F. (1982). Onset of depressive psychiatric crises and the menstrual cycle. *Am. J. Psychiatry*, **139**, 475–8.

Alves, S.E., Weiland, N.G., Hayashi, S. & McEwen, B.S. (1998). Immunocytochemical localization of nuclear estrogen receptors and progestin receptors within the rat dorsal raphe nucleus. *J. Compr. Neurol.*, **391**, 322–4.

Angermeyer, M.C. & Kuhn, L. (1988). Gender differences in age at onset of schizophrenia, an overview. *Eur. Arch. Psychiatry Neurol. Sci.*, **237**, 351–4.

Anis-Ur-Rehman, St Clair, D. & Platz, C. (1990). Puerperal insanity in the 19th and 20th centuries. *Br. J. Psychiatry*, **156**, 861–5.

Behrens, S., Hafner, H., De Vry, J. & Gattaz, W.F. (1992). Estradiol attenuates dopamine-medicated behaviour in rats. Implications for sex differences in schizophrenia. *Schizophr. Res.*, **6**, 114.

Berlin, F.S., Berger, G.K. & Morey, J. (1982). Periodic psychosis of puberty: a case report. *Am. J. Psychiatry*, **139**, 119–20.

Brambilla, F. & Penati, G. (1978). Perspectives in endocrine psychobiology. *Perspectives in Endocrine Psychobiology* ed. F. Brambilla & P. Bridges, pp. 309–422. London: G.J. Witey.

Clopton, J. & Gordon, J.H. (1986). In vivo effects of estrogen and 2-hydroxy estradiol on D-2 dopamine receptor agonist affinity states in rate striatum. *J. Neural Transmiss.*, **66**, 13–20.

Cone, R.I., Davis, G.A. & Coy, R.W. (1981). Effects of ovarian steroids on serotonin metabolism within grossly dissected and microdissected brain regions of the ovariectomized rat. *Brain Res. Bull.*, **7**, 639–44.

Dalton, K. (1959). Menstruation and acute psychiatric illness. *Br. Med. J.*, **1**, 148–9.

Dalton, K. (1980). *Depression after Childbirth.* Oxford: Oxford University Press.

Dennerstein, L., Judd, F. & Davies, B. (1983). Psychosis and the menstrual cycle. *Med. J. Aust.*, **1**, 524–6.

Di Paolo, T., Payet, P. & Labrie, F. (1982). Effect of prolactin and estradiol on rat striated dopamine receptors. *Life Sci.*, **31**, 2921–9.

Endo, M., Daiguji, M., Asano, Y., Yanashita, I. & Lakahashi, S. (1978). Periodic psychosis occurring in association with the menstrual cycle. *J. Clin. Psychiatry*, **39**, 456–61.

Felthous, A.R., Robinson, D.B. & Conroy, R.W. (1980). Prevention of recurrent menstrual psychosis by an oral contraceptive. *Am. J. Psychiatry*, **137**, 245–6.

Ferretti, C., Blengio, M., Vigna, I., Ghia, P. & Gerazzani, E. (1992). Effects of estradiol on the ontogenesis of striatial dopamine D_1 and D_2 receptor sites in male and female rats. *Brain Res.*, **571**, 212–17.

Fink, G. (1995). The psychoprotective action of estrogen is mediated by central serotonergic as well as dopaminergic mechanisms. In *Serotonin in the Central Nervous System and Periphery* ed. A. Takada & G. Curzon, pp. 175–87. Holland: Elsevier Science BV.

Fink, G., Sumner, B., McQueen, J.K., Wilson, H. & Rose, R. (1998). Sex steroid control of mood, mental state and memory. *Clin. Exp. Pharmacol. Physiol.*, **25**, pp. 764–5.

Fink, G., Sumner, B., Rosie, R., Wilson, H. & McQueen, J. (1999). Androgen actions on central serotonin neurotransmission: relevance for mood, mental state and memory. *Behav. Brain Res.*, **105**, 53–68.

George, A.J. & Sandler, M. (1988). Endocrine and biochemical studies in puerperal mental disorders. In *Motherhood and Mental Illness 2 – Causes and Consequences*, ed. R. Kumar & I.F. Brockington. London: Butterworth.

George, A.J. & Wilson, K.C.M. (1982). Maternal beta-endorphin/beta-lipotrophin immunoreactivity correlates with maternal prolactin in the first postpartum week. *Br. J. Clin. Pharmacol.*, **14**, 146–7.

George, A.J., Copeland, J.R.M. & Wilson, K.C.M. (1980). Serum prolaction and the post-partum blues syndrome. *Br. J. Pharmacol.*, **70**, 102–3.

Gordon, J.H. & Perry, K.O. (1983). Pre- and postsynaptic neurochemical alteration following estrogen-induced striatal dopamine hypo- and hypersensitivity. *Brain Res. Bull.*, **10**, 425–8.

Gordon, J.H., Borison, R.L. & Diamond, B.I. (1980). Modulation of dopamine receptor sensitivity by estrogen. *Biol. Psychiatry*, **15**, 389–96.

Hackmann, E., Wirz-Justice, A. & Lichtsteiner, M. (1973). The uptake of dopamine and serotonin in rat brain during progesterone decline. *Psychopharmacologia*, **32**, 183–91.

Hafner, H. (1991). The epidemiology of beginning schizophrenia. Presented at the WPA section of epidemiology and community psychiatry symposium. Oslo, June 14–16.

Hafner, H., Riecher, A., Maurer, K. et al. (1990). Instrument for the Retrospective Assessment of the Onset of Schizophrenia – IRAOS. *Z. Klin. Psychol.*, **19**, 230–55.

Hafner, H., Maurer, K., Loffler, W., an der Heiden, W., Munk-Jorgensen, P., Hambrecht, M. & Reicher-Rossler, A. (1998). The ABC schizophrenia study: a preliminary overview of the results. *Soc. Psychiatry Psychiatr. Epidemiol.*, **33**, 380–6.

Hallonquist, J.D., Seeman, M.V., Lang, M. & Rector, N.A. (1993). Variation in symptom severity over the menstrual cycle of schizophrenics. *Bio. Psychiatry*, **33**, 207–9.

Hambrecht, M., Maurer, K., Hafner, H. & Sartorius, N. (1992). Transnational stability of gender differences in schizophrenia? An analysis based on the WHO study on determinants of outcome of severe mental disorders. *Eur. Arch. Psychiatry Clin. Neurosci.*, **242**, 6–12.

Hatotani, N., Nishikubo, M. & Kitayama, I. (1959). Periodic psychoses in the female and the reproductive process. In *Psychoneuro-endocrinology in Reproduction*, ed. L. Zichella & P. Panchevi, pp. 55–68. Amsterdam: Elsevier.

Hoskins, R.G. (1929). Endocrine factors in dementia praecox. *N. Engl. J. Med.*, **200**, 361.

Hruska, R.E., Ludmer, L.M. & Silbergeld, E.K. (1980). Hypophysectomy prevents the striatal dopamine receptor supersensitivity produced by chronic haloperidol treatment. *Eur. J. Pharmacol.*, **65**, 455–6.

Joyce, J.N., Smith, R.L. & Van Hartesveldt, C. (1982). Estradiol suppresses then enhances intracaudate dopamine-induced contralateral deviation. *Eur. J. Pharm.*, **81**, 117–22.

Kane, F.J. (1985). Postpartum disorders. In *Psychiatry IV*, ed. H. Kaplan & B. Saddock, pp. 1238–41. Baltimore: Williams & Wilkins.

Kathol, R.G., Gehris, T.L., Carroll, B.T. et al. (1992). Blunted ACTH response to hypoglycemic stress in depressed patients but not in patients with schizophrenia. *J. Psychiatry Res.*, **26**, 103–16.

Kay, S.R., Fiszbein, A. & Opler, L.A. (1987). The Positive and Negative Syndrome Scale (PANSS) for schizophrenia. *Schizophr. Bull.*, **13**, 261–7.

Keks, N., Copolov, D. & Singh, B. (1987). Abnormal prolactin response to haloperidol challenge in men with schizophrenia. *Am. J. Psychiatry*, **144**, 1335–7.

Kraepelin, E. (1892). *Psychiatrie*, vol. 3, part 2, 8th edn. Translated (1919). *Dementia Praecox and Paraphrenia*. Edinburgh: Livingstone.

Kraepelin, E. (1909–15). *Psychiatre*, vols. 1–4. Leipzig: Barth.

Kuevi, V., Carson, R. & Dixson, A.F. (1983). Plasma amine and hormone changes in 'post partum blues'. *Clin. Endocrinol.*, **19**, 39–46.

Kulkarni, J., de Castella, A., Smith, D., Taffe, J., Keks, N. & Copolov, D. (1996a). A clinical trial of the effects of estrogen in acutely psychotic women. *Schizophr. Res.*, **20**, 247–52.

Kulkarni, J., Gostt, K & de Castella, A. (1996b). The menstrual cycle in women with schizophrenia. *Schizophr. Res.* **18**, 254.

Kumar, R., Isaac, S. & Meltzer, E. (1983). Recurrent postpartum psychosis: a model for prospective clinical investigation. *Br. J. Psychiatry*, **142**, 618–20.

Lerer, B., Ran, A., Blacker, M. et al. (1988). Neuroendocrine responses in chronic schizophrenia. *Schizophr. Res.*, **1**, 405–10.

Lewine, R. (1988). Gender and schizophrenia. In *Handbook of Schizophrenia*, ed. M.T. Tsuang & J.C. Simpson, pp. 379–97. Amsterdam: Elsevier.

Lieberman, J.A. & Koreen, A.R. (1993). Neurochemistry and neuroendocrinology of schizophrenia: a selective review. *Schizophr. Bull.*, **19**, 371–429.

Lingjaerde, P. & Bredland, R. (1954). Hyperestrogenic cyclic psychosis. *Acta Psychiatr. Neurol. Scand.*, **29**, 355–60.

Luggin, R., Bernsted, L., Petersson, B. & Jacobsen, A.T. (1984). Acute psychiatric admission related to the menstrual cycle. *Acta Psychiatr. Scand.*, **69**, 461–5.

Mason, J.W. (1975). Emotion as reflected in patterns of endocrine investigation. In *Emotions; Their Parameters and Measurement* ed. L Levi, pp. 143–81. New York: Raven Press.

McEwen, B.S., Biegon, A., Rainbow, T.C., Paden, C., Snyder, L. & DeGroff, V. (1981). The interaction of estrogens with intracellular receptors and with putative neurotransmitter receptors: implications for the mechanisms of activation of regulation of sexual behaviour and ovulation. In *Steroid Hormone Regulation of the Brain*, ed. K Fuxe, J.A. Gustafsson & L. Wetterberg, pp. 15–29. New York: Pergammon Press.

Moos, R.F. (1968). The development of a menstrual distress questionnaire. *Psychosom. Med.*, **6**, 853–67.

Mosselman, S., Polman, J. & Dukema, R. (1996). ER beta: identification and characterization of a novel human estrogen receptor. *FEBS Lett.*, **392**, 49–53.

Newham, J.P., Dennett, P.M. & Ferron, S.A. (1984). A study of the relationship between circulating beta-endorphin-like immunoreactivity and post-partum 'blues'. *J. Clin. Endocrinol.*, **20**, 169–77.

Nickelsen, T., Lufkin, E.G., Riggs, B.L., Cox, D.A. & Crook, T.H. (1999). Raloxifene hydrochoride, a selective estrogen receptor modulator: safety assessment of effects on cognitive function and mood in postmenopausal women. *Pscyhoneuroendocrinology*, **24**, 115–28.

Nott, P.N., Frankslin, M., Armitage, C. & Gelder, M.G. (1976). Hormonal changes in mood in the puerperium. *Br. J. Psychiatry*, **128**, 379–83.

Overall, J.E. & Gorham, D.R. (1962). The brief psychiatric rating scale. *Psychol. Rep.*, **10**, 799–812.

Perry, K.O., Diamond, B.I., Fields, J.Z. & Gordon, J.H. (1981). Hypophysectomy induced hypersensitivity to dopamine: antagonism by estrogen. *Brain Res.*, **226**, 211–19.

Riecher-Rossler, A., Hafner, H., Maurer, K., Stummbaum, M. & Schmidt, R. (1992). Schizophrenic symptomatology varies with serum estradiol levels during menstrual cycle. *Schizophr. Res.*, **6**, 114–15.

Riecher-Rossler, A., Hafner, H., Stumnbaum, M., Maurer, K. & Schmidt, R. (1994). Can estradiol modulate schizophrenic symptomatology? *Schizophr. Bull.*, **20**, 203–13.

Rosen, G. (1968). *Madness in Society*. London: Routledge.

Sachar, E.J., Mason, J.W., Kolmer, H.S. & Arfess, K.L. (1963). Psychoendocrine aspects of acute schizophrenic reactions. *Psychosom. Med.*, **25**, 510.

Scot, R. (1534). In: *The Discovery of Witchcraft*. (1972). New York: Centaur Press.

Seeman, M.V. (1983). Interaction of sex, age and neuroleptic dose. *Compr. Psychiatry*, **24**, 125–8.

Seeman, M.V. & Lang, M. (1990). The role of estrogens in schizophrenia gender differences. *Schizophr. Bull.*, **16**, 185–95.

Shughrue, P.J., Lane, M.V. & Merchenthaler, I. (1997). Comparative distribution of estrogen receptor and X and B MRNA in the rat central nervous system. *J. Compr. Neurol.*, **388**, 507–25.

Solthau, A. & Taylor, R. (1982). Depression after childbirth. *Br. Med. J.*, **284**, 980–1.

Sumner, B.E.H., Grant, K.E., Rosie, R., Hegele-Hartung, Ch., Fritzemeier, K.-H. & Fink, G. (1999). Effects of tamoxifen on serotonin transporter and 5-hydroxytryptamine $_{2A}$ receptor binding sites and mRNA levels in the brain of ovariectomized rats with or without acute estradiol replacement. *Mol. Brain Res.*, **73**, 119–28.

Torghele, J. (1957). Premenstrual tension in psychotic women. *Lancet*, **ii**, 163–70.

Vogel, P., Soddu, G., Reicher, A. & Gattaz, W.F. (1992). Effects of the menstrual cycle on therapeutic response in schizophrenic patients. *Schizophr. Res.*, **6**, 115.

Wieck, A., Kumar, R., Hirst, A.D., Marks, M.N., Campbell, I.C. & Checkley, S.A. (1991). Increased sensitivity of dopamine receptors and recurrence of affective psychosis after childbirth. *Br. Med. J.*, **303**, 613–16.

Zola, P., Meyerson, A. T., Reznikoff, M., Thornton, J. C. & Concool, B. M. (1979). Menstrual symptomatology and psychiatric admission. *J. Psychosom. Res.*, **23**, 241–5.

6

Reproductive, preconceptual and antenatal needs of women with schizophrenia

Joanne Barkla and John McGrath

Many women with schizophrenia are or will become mothers. Their transition into parenthood can be problematic due to the illness itself as well as to the many psychosocial difficulties associated with chronic mental illness. In this chapter we provide a selective review of the literature about the special needs of women with schizophrenia in the areas of family planning and antenatal care. There is a growing awareness that good antenatal care starts before conception. Clinicians involved in the care of women with schizophrenia who are in their reproductive years should include these issues routinely in their assessments and treatment plans. There is a special need to improve antenatal services for women with schizophrenia in light of the growing evidence that the offspring of these women are at increased risk of obstetric complications. The reader is also referred to Chapter 7, which examines motherhood and schizophrenia, and to Chapter 8, which concentrates on treatment aspects of schizophrenia in women.

Reproductive issues for women with schizophrenia

A number of authors (Odegard, 1980; Miller et al., 1992) have suggested that the rate of pregnancy amongst those with chronic schizophrenia has increased since deinstitutionalization. This may be as a direct result of increased availability of sexual partners, or concurrent changing attitudes towards conception amongst those with serious mental illness.

Of those with schizophrenia and related disorders, women are more likely then men to be involved in parenting and to be living with a member of the opposite sex (Test et al., 1990). In Miller & Finnerty's (1996) study of sexuality, reproduction and child rearing, women who had diagnoses of either schizophrenia or schizoaffective disorder were more likely than women without illness to have had more than one sexual partner. They were also more likely to have a negative sexual experience, to have been raped or have been in receipt of payment for sex. Both groups showed similar birth rates and espoused similar attitudes towards pregnancy. Women with chronic mental illness have also been shown to have a high incidence of unplanned and unwanted pregnancies (Coverdale et al., 1993; Miller & Finnerty, 1996).

Pregnancy

A number of developmental tasks have been described for women making the transition from pregnancy to motherhood. These include the mother's degree of acceptance of the pregnancy, affiliation with the fetus, preparatory behaviour and the development of a reality-based perception of the neonate (Cohen, 1993). In women with schizophrenia these tasks may be impeded not only by the psychotic experiences themselves, but also by associated negative influences such as previous loss of custody of infants or poor social support.

A number of theories have been proposed to try to explain the impact of pregnancy on women. These include biological, psychodynamic and developmental, and the diathesis/stress models. Risk factors which have been associated with poor postnatal adjustment include: a history of previous psychiatric illness; physiological and biological factors such as those relating to the type of delivery; previous gynaecological dysfunction; personality and attitudes of the mother; psychosocial variables; stressful life events; marital disharmony; and infant temperament. The presence of a psychotic illness frequently attracts additional stressors and is often itself associated with poorer social supports, single parenthood and varying combinations of those factors mentioned above.

Sociodemographic characteristics

Women with serious mental illness are more likely to be without the support of a spouse or significant other, to have had an unplanned pregnancy, and to hold a negative attitude towards their pregnancy (McNeil et al., 1983; Rudolph et al., 1990). McNeil and colleagues (1983), for example, found that only 26% of women with a past history of non-organic psychosis had experienced the triad of a planned pregnancy, supportive relationship with the infant's father and good support from significant family members. A review by Rudolph et al. (1990) of 35 pregnant women receiving inpatient treatment for psychotic disorders found high rates of separation, divorce and being without the support of significant others. Of the 35 subjects, five had been homeless and many had not been in receipt of treatment prior to admission. The sample was drawn from inpatients, and these findings may not generalize to all pregnant women with psychotic illnesses. Miller (1990) found that 36% of 57 pregnant women admitted to a psychiatric hospital had previously been homeless.

In an Australian study, 62% of women with a psychotic illness who had been referred to an obstetric consultation liaison service were unmarried (Dunsis & Smith, 1996). Zemencuk et al. (1995) reported that poorer education, a diagnosis of schizophrenia and an early age of illness onset were associated with pregnancy at a younger age.

Course of illness during pregnancy

The evidence regarding the impact of pregnancy on the course of schizophrenia is conflicting, possibly reflecting how variable the impact of pregnancy is, depending not only on diagnosis but also on a range of psychological and social variables. It may also be a result of a methodologically diverse array of studies, often using small sample sizes.

Bagedahl-Strindlund (1986) surveyed women who had given birth during 1976 and 1977 in County Stockholm and who had had a psychiatric admission between 20 weeks' gestation and the end of the first postpartum year. The most significant risk time for relapse of psychosis was within 3 months postpartum, and especially within 1 month. No association was found between sociodemographic factors and the time of onset of illness. Marital discord was more frequent in women who had had an onset of illness during pregnancy itself.

McNeil et al. (1984) found that in those women with a history of a psychotic disorder, a worsening of symptoms during pregnancy was more common than improvement in mental state. In contrast, women without a history of psychotic disorder experienced only minor changes in mental state during pregnancy. Pregnancy seemingly has an unpredictable and highly variable impact on mental health and the effect of pregnancy cannot be predicted by mental state in the 6 months before conception. Amongst those with serious mental illness, age and the effect of the pregnancy on physical health are the only variables found to have been of statistical significance. McNeil and colleagues (1984) concluded that the factors which contribute to a woman's mental health during pregnancy are complex and that if there are any significant factors they may be too varied or unsystematic to measure, or be at a biological or intrapsychic level not assessed in the study.

There is more general consensus that the postpartum period represents a time when mothers with a history of psychotic illness, especially affective psychosis (Brockington et al., 1982), are particularly vulnerable (see Chapters 5 and 7). Kumar et al. (1995) prospectively studied 100 consecutive admissions to a mother-and-baby unit and found that the majority of women with a history of bipolar affective disorder relapsed within 2 weeks of childbirth. Women with schizophrenia were less likely to have acute episodes but rather a continuation of chronic symptoms throughout the pregnancy and postpartum period. Three of the 20 women with diagnoses of schizophrenia experienced an exacerbation of symptoms. However, most of them (60%) were also admitted within the 2-week period after the birth of their child. Of the mothers with schizophrenia, 50% were separated from their infants at discharge and, in all but one case, fostering or adoption became permanent. The fact that only 30% of mothers had a current partner, and over a third were discharged to a supervisory setting may have contributed to this outcome.

Impact of psychosis on pregnancy

Miller (1990) has discussed the occurrence and significance of specific symptoms such as denial of pregnancy in women with psychotic disorders. Those who experience psychotic denial are more likely to have schizophrenia, and to have lost custody of children. Most of these women with schizophrenia anticipate the loss of their child. Those who expect to lose their child are more likely to deny their pregnancy. Miller (1990) also reported that many women with schizophrenia have their attachment to their offspring compromised by the realities of their psychosocial situation and the likelihood that they would be unable to care for the child. Thus, these women appear at times to be denying the problems facing them and holding idealized fantasies of nurturing their children. Miller noted that ambivalent feelings towards the father of the infant were precipitants for psychotic denial. The implication of psychotic denial for the mother and her infant is that they are at increased risk of non-compliance with antenatal care, a precipitous delivery and, rarely, infanticide.

As Miller & Finnerty (1996) and other authors have recognized, there is a need to include in the treatment of women with serious mental illness topics such as sex education, social skills and assertiveness training. These women need screening for sexually transmitted diseases, advice on family planning and facilitated access to antenatal care (see also Chapter 8).

In addition to denial, the diagnosis of pregnancy may be delayed because of poor self-observation, or fear and suspicion of health professionals. Women with psychotic disorders may make distorted interpretations of the changes and experiences associated with pregnancy (Spielvogel & Wile, 1986). Those with schizophrenia may experience an intensification of delusional ideas precipitated by fetal movement and may be ambivalent towards the pregnancy. They may have difficulty cooperating with antenatal procedures.

In Miller's (1990) review of 57 pregnant patients on a psychiatric ward, 34% had made or planned a suicide attempt before admission. Substance abuse was reported in 64% of these women. In a later study, Miller & Finnerty (1996) found similar rates of drug use in a group of women with psychosis, compared to women without psychosis and likewise, similar attempts to reduce drug use during pregnancy. The women with psychotic disorders were also more likely to have been victims of violence whilst pregnant, and were less likely to have received prenatal care (only 73.5% reported that they had).

Antenatal care and the primary prevention of schizophrenia

In the field of schizophrenia research, there is a convergence of several streams of evidence that support the neurodevelopmental hypothesis. This hypothesis proposes an early disturbance of brain development which causes a lifelong disorder whose signs and symptoms change over time as a function of the maturity of the central nervous system (Lewis & Murray, 1987). In adult life, the consequence of this early brain lesion is the clinical disorder schizophrenia. There is considerable evidence that perinatal difficulties are a part of the complex of factors that contribute to the aetiology of a proportion of cases of schizophrenia (McNeil & Kaij, 1978; Geddes & Lawrie, 1995; McGrath & Murray, 1995). Genetically predisposed fetuses apparently have a special vulnerability that amplifies the damage which perinatal complications inflict on their brains (Mednick et al., 1987).

One interesting implication of these findings is the possibility that intensive intervention in the gestation of high-risk fetuses may reduce the likelihood of obstetric complications, thus reducing a potential risk factor for schizophrenia in the offspring. Interventions that optimize fetal neurodevelopment and reduce birth complications may serve as a buffer to protect the vulnerable fetus. Factors amenable to intervention (e.g. compliance with antenatal attendance, stop-smoking programmes and nutritional advice) warrant investigation in this particular population. Furthermore, there is considerable (but not incontrovertible) evidence that general social support has an impact on obstetric variables. Oakley (1985) in her influential review commented: 'It is concluded that there is considerable evidence to suggest that intervention programs aimed at improving the "social side" of antenatal care are capable of affecting birthweight and other "hard" measures of pregnancy outcomes' (p. 1265). However, this area is plagued by methodological problems, and a full discussion of these issues is outside the scope of this review.

A recent paper from Crow's group (Sacker et al., 1996) describes a meta-analysis of data examining whether the offspring of women with psychosis experienced more obstetric complications. They found that the offspring of psychotic women did experience more preganancy and birth complications than controls and had lower birth weight and poorer neonatal condition.

In light of the paucity of background information on pregnant women who have a serious mental illness, and in view of the potential avenues for primary prevention, we propose that special attention be given to this group. There is mounting evidence that optimal antenatal care may have long-term benefits for the fetus as well as for the mother. Regardless of these speculations, in order to provide optimal support for parents with mental illness, the mother should be linked to appropriate services at the earliest opportunity. This will allow for the organization of the various services that would assist the parent after the birth – a time of particular vulnerability for the mother as well as the offspring.

Women with schizophrenia tend to have poor attendance records at antenatal clinics (Miller, 1990), and thus have less opportunity for review of their health and less access to education regarding pregnancy and parenting. In Miller's (1990) review of a population of psychiatric inpatients, 48% were non-compliant with antenatal appointments after discharge from hospital. Those who were non-compliant were on average older and were more likely to be unemployed and without permanent residence. They also had a higher rate of unplanned pregnancies, and were more likely to have had a psychotic presentation.

Despite this, women with psychosis may be more likely to seek antenatal help during pregnancy than attend a mental health clinic, particularly for acute antenatal care (Krener et al., 1989). A contributory factor may be the fear that they may be encouraged by psychiatric staff to undergo a termination of pregnancy. This presents a window of opportunity for mental health services to intervene through the antenatal services.

Consideration should be given to system-related factors such as over-crowding, long waiting times, lack of continuity of care and transport to and from clinics, which may deter women from seeking care. Other factors which may influence whether women attend are attitudinal factors, such as having an unplanned pregnancy, an indifferent attitude to antenatal care, poor social supports and failure to recognize signs of pregnancy (Brown, 1989).

There is a lack of evidence on the efficacy of antenatal programmes designed for women with schizophrenia. There is, however, compelling evidence supporting the benefits of good antenatal care for high-risk groups. It remains unclear whether this can be generalized to those women with schizophrenia, as the mechanism by which their risk is increased remains speculative. Some evidence supports the notion that prolonged hospitalization for women with schizophrenia during pregnancy improves the outcome (Muqtadir et al., 1986); the downsides to this include dislocation from family and society and the possibility of dependence and institutionalization.

Whilst many authors recommended increasing support for education and parenting classes, there are few studies looking at the impact of these interventions on the ability of the mother to care for her infant.

Preconceptual counselling

The risk associated with an unplanned pregnancy and the need for education about family planning is particularly evident amongst women with serious mental illness. The first 8 weeks of gestation are critical for fetal neural development and the brain is highly susceptible to teratogenic agents during this period of embryonic life. An unplanned pregnancy minimizes the opportunity to prepare and optimize conditions for the fetus from the time of conception. These women may be on a variety of medications, smoking heavily and using illicit substances. By virtue of poor social circumstance or poverty, they may not be meeting adequate nutritional requirements. In addition, adjustment to pregnancy and parenthood may be compromised by an unwanted pregnancy. It is possible that these factors will impact on a mother's compliance with antenatal care, her ability to parent and her mental state.

One might expect that, parallel to changing social attitudes, there would be increased availability, knowledge and use of contraception amongst women with psychotic disorders. However, these factors may not have had an impact on the population of women and men with psychiatric illness to the same extent as it has on the general community. Coverdale et al. (1993), in their study of 82 clinic-based health professionals, found that although the health workers recognized the importance of family planning, they had raised the issue with only 25% of their patients. Only 10% of their female patients confirmed that family planning had been discussed with them. The inconvenience and problematic side-effects of some contraceptives cannot be ignored in this population of women any more than they can in those women who do not have serious mental illness. McCullough et al. (1992) have highlighted the need for contraception to be effective and have pointed out that the disorganization which may occur in women with schizophrenia can result in barrier methods and oral contraceptives not being used reliably. Depot preparations may offer more reliable contraception.

Coverdale et al. (1997) recommended that, in developing family planning for women with psychosis, an emphasis should be placed on taking a thorough sexual history. This includes eliciting information that will reveal whether the woman may already be pregnant, particularly as there is a risk that she might deny the pregnancy; whether she might be at risk of having an unwanted pregnancy; or whether she is at risk of a sexually transmitted disease. A thorough review of previous pregnancies and an assessment of the ability to mother children, should be included.

As Miller & Finnerty (1996) and other authors have recognized, there is a need to include in the treatment of women with serious mental illness topics such as sex education, social skills and assertiveness training. These women need screening for sexually transmitted diseases, advice on family planning and facilitated access to antenatal care. There should be integration with other important services such as parenting classes and services for prevention of sexually transmitted diseases.

Consideration is needed as to where education takes place. The advantages of it occurring within the mental health service include having staff who may have a better understanding of the difficulties these women have in learning and understanding. Health workers who have less experience with the mentally ill may feel less confident in discussing these issues with them. Coverdale et al. (1993) support the integration of such services and incorporating them with parenting classes. Such integration may also increase the number of women being reached.

The need for guidelines for preconception counselling, management and care of pregnant women with medical conditions such as epilepsy have been well recognized. Perhaps some of these principles should equally apply to women with schizophrenia.

In summary, it is reasonable to suggest that women with schizophrenia should be assisted in avoiding unwanted pregnancies but those who do fall pregnant should be given optimal support to carry wanted pregnancies to term (Abernethy & Grunebaum, 1972). Addressing contraception and suitability to have custody of the child in this population and liaison between disciplines will contribute to comprehensive care for the mother and her infant (Rudolph et al., 1990).

Ethical considerations

Complex ethical and legal issues may arise in dealing with contraception and antenatal care for women with schizophrenia. When contraception is decided upon, it must be effective, and consideration should be given to difficulties with compliance for women who are psychiatrically unwell. The rights of the woman to be a mother need to be respected and staff must be mindful of the ability of the woman to give continuing, informed consent. The health of the fetus and the child also need to be incorporated into the management plan. Regarding treatment of women with serious mental illness during pregnancy, Miller et al. (1992) have also raised the question of whether pregnancy itself should play a role in the decision whether to admit women against their will to psychiatric facilities. Certainly, if compulsory admission is to be used to improve perinatal outcome, inpatient and outpatient settings must incorporate appropriate antenatal services (Miller et al., 1992).

Conclusions

The majority of women with schizophrenia will become mothers. This has implications for service development and the need to provide appropriate and timely interventions for this group of women. It is possible that, through improving collaboration between services and provision of additional supports, there is the potential to reduce maternal morbidity and possibly for primary prevention of psychiatric morbidity in the offspring. Hence, we may be better able to assist women with schizophrenia with their transition into motherhood, to assist them in optimizing the conditions for parenting, or support them through the loss if they are unwilling or unable to parent their infant.

REFERENCES

Abernethy, V.D. & Grunebaum, H. (1972). Toward a family planning program in psychiatric hospitals. *Am. J. Public Health*, **62**, 1638–46.

Bagedahl-Strindlund, M. (1986). Postpartum mental illness: timing of illness onset and the relation to symptoms and sociodemographic characteristics. *Acta Psychiatr. Scand.*, **74** 490–6.

Brockington, I.F., Perris, C., Kendell, R.W., Hillier, V.E. & Wainwright, S. (1982). The course and outcome of cycloid psychosis. *Psychol. Med.*, **12**, 91–105.

Brown, S.S. (1989). Drawing women into prenatal care. *Fam. Plann. Perspect.*, **21**, 73–80.

Cohen, C.I. (1993). Poverty and the course of schizophrenia: implications for research and policy. *Hosp. Commun. Psychiatry*, **44**, 951–8.

Coverdale, J.H., Bayer, T.L., McCullough, L.B. & Chervenak, F.A. (1993). Respecting the autonomy of chronic mentally ill women in decisions about contraception. *Hosp. Commun. Psychiatry*, **44**, 671–4.

Coverdale, J.H., Turbott, S.H. & Roberts, H. (1997). Family planning needs and STD risk behaviours of female psychiatric out-patients. *Br. J. Psychiatry*, **171**, 69–72.

Dunsis, A. & Smith, G.C. (1996). Consultation liaison psychiatry in an obstetric service. *Aust. N.Z. J. Psychiatry*, **30**, 63–73.

Geddes, J.R. & Lawrie, S.M. (1995). Obstetric complications and schizophrenia: a meta-analysis. *Br. J. Psychiatry*, **167**, 786–93.

Krener, P., Simmons, M.K., Hansen, R.L. & Treat, J.N. (1989). Effect of pregnancy on psychosis: life circumstances and psychiatric symptoms. *Int. J. Psychiatr. Med.*, **19**, 65–84.

Kumar, R., Marks, M., Platz, C. & Yoshida, K. (1995). Clinical survey of a psychiatric mother and baby: characteristics of 100 consecutive admissions. *J. Affect. Dis.*, **33**, 11–22.

Lewis, S.W. & Murray, R.M. (1987). Obstetric complications, neurodevelopmental deviance, and risk of schizophrenia. *J. Psychiatr. Res.*, **21**, 413–21.

McCullough, L.B., Coverdale, J., Bayer, T. & Chervenak, F.A. (1992). Ethically justified guidelines for family planning interventions to prevent pregnancy planning in female patients with a chronic mental illness. *Am. J. Obstet. Gynecol*, **167**, 19–25.

McGrath, J.J. & Murray, R.M. (1995). Risk factors for schizophrenia: from conception to birth. In *Schizophrenia*, ed. D.R. Weinberger, & S.R. Hirsch, pp. 187–205. Oxford: Blackwells.

McNeil, T.F. & Kaij, L. (1978). Obstetric factors in the development of schizophrenia: complications in the births of preschizophrenics and in reproductions by schizophrenic parents. In *The Nature of Schizophrenia: New Approaches to Research and Treatment.* ed. L.C. Wynne, R.L. Cromwell & S. Matthysse, pp. 401–29. New York: John Wiley.

McNeil, T.F., Kaij, L., Malmquist, L.A. et al. (1983). Offspring of women with nonorganic psychoses. Development of a longitudinal study of children at high risk. *Acta Psychiatr. Scand.*, **68**, 234–50.

McNeil, T.F., Kaij, L. & Malmquiat-Larsson, A. (1984). Women with nonorganic psychosis: pregnancy's effect on mental health during pregnancy. Obstetric complications in schizophrenic patients. *Acta Psychiatr. Scand.*, **70**, 140–8.

Mednick, S.A., Parnas, J. & Schulsinger, F. (1987). The Copenhagen high-risk project, 1962–86. *Schizophr. Bull.*, **13**, 485–95.

Miller, L.J. (1990). Psychotic denial of pregnancy: phenomenology and clinical management. *Hosp. Commun. Psychiatry*, **41**, 1233–7.

Miller, L.J. & Finnerty, M. (1996). Sexuality, pregnancy, and childbearing among women with schizophrenia-spectrum disorders. *Psychiatr. Serv.*, **47**, 502–6.

Miller, W.H., Bloom, J.D. & Resnick, M.P. (1992). Prenatal care for pregnant chronic mentally ill patients. *Hosp. Commun. Psychiatry*, **43**, 942–3.

Muqtadir, S., Hamann, M.W. & Molnar, G. (1986). Management of psychotic pregnant patients in a medical–psychiatric unit. *Psychosomatics*, **27**, 31–3.

Oakley, A. (1985). Social support in pregnancy: the 'soft' way to increase birthweight? *Soc. Sci. Med.*, **21**, 1259–68.

Odegard, O. (1980). Fertility of psychiatric first admissions in Norway 1936–1975. *Acta Psychiatr. Scand.*, **62**, 212–20.

Rudolph, B., Larson, G.L., Sweeny, S., Hough, E.E. & Arorian, K. (1990). Hospitalized pregnant psychotic women: characteristics and treatment issues. *Hosp. Commun. Psychiatry*, **41**, 159–63.

Sacker, A., Done, D.J. & Crow, T.J. (1996). Obstetric complications in children born to parents with schizophrenia: a meta-analysis of case control studies. *Psychol. Med.*, **26**, 279–87.

Spielvogel, J. & Wile, J. (1986). Treatment of the psychotic pregnant patient. *Psychosomatics*, **27**, 487–92.

Test, S.A., Burke, S.S. & Wallisch, L.S. (1990). Gender differences of young adults with schizophrenic disorders in community care. *Schizophr. Bull.*, **16**, 331–44.

Zemencuk, J., Rogosch, F.A. & Mowbray, C.T. (1995). The seriously mentally ill woman in the role of parent: characteristics, parenting sensitivity, and needs. *Psychol. Rehab. J.*, **18**, 72–92.

7

Motherhood and schizophrenia

Jenny Hearle and John McGrath

In this chapter we discuss selected topics related to motherhood and schizophrenia. We examine the number of women with schizophrenia who are mothers, in order to define the extent of the issue. Drawing on a recent Australian study, we further explore the links between motherhood and schizophrenia, addressing issues such as when women with schizophrenia have their children with respect to the onset of their illness. The second part of the chapter focuses on more practical issues, such as what type of help parents with psychotic disorders receive in caring for their children, and what barriers exist to such assistance. Finally, we make recommendations aimed at improving intersectorial liaison.

Mothers with schizophrenia, as parents

People with serious mental illness have the same aspirations for parenthood and face the same challenges associated with parenthood as other community members (Sand, 1995). Marriage and motherhood are expected milestones in life for most women, marking the transition to adulthood and often accompanied by special rites and ceremonies. Motherhood in particular is a valued social role in every human society. The right to bear children and parent them is identified as a basic human right under United Nations agreements. Reproduction is regarded as a fundamental right in our society and may not be denied on the basis of disability alone.

For some women with schizophrenia, motherhood results in improved social networks, reduced feelings of identity confusion and stigma and a meaningful work role (Schwab et al., 1991). For others, however, motherhood is associated with grief, loss and frustration (Human Rights and

Equal Opportunity Commission, 1993). The stigma associated with serious mental illness appears to be amplified when it comes to parents with mental illness. Research in Australia has examined attitudes to mental illness in the general community (Reark Research, 1993, unpublished data). Based on random-digit telephone dialling, 1224 Australians were interviewed about their knowledge of and attitudes to a broad range of mental health issues. In response to the statement 'Even if they seem all right, it is better for people who've had a mental illness not to have children', 21% of respondents either agreed or strongly agreed; a further 14% were neutral (neither agreed nor disagreed). Men were more likely to agree with the statement, especially those over 55 years (44% in agreement with the statement). This high level of stigma adds an extra layer of stress and anxiety to the new mother.

Previous research relating to schizophrenia and parenthood has largely focused on the identification of risk factors that may adversely impact on the child. Children of parents with serious mental illness, who have an increased risk of developing mental illness due to genetic factors, show higher rates of behavioural and emotional disorders (Goodman, 1984; Rutter & Quinton, 1984). Often the literature presents a negative view in relation to parental mental illness, with a tendency to portray parents as 'toxic' or dangerous towards their offspring (Oates, 1977). In contrast, there is only a small body of research that focuses on the positive and health-promoting aspects of parenthood for people with serious mental illness (Mowbray et al., 1997).

The impact of a mentally ill parent on family functioning is mediated via complex interactions including illness-related factors (e.g. core symptoms of the illness, side-effects of medication and need for hospitalization) and secondary psychosocial factors (e.g. impaired parenting skills, marital discord, social isolation, insecure and poor housing, unemployment and poverty; Dohrenwend & Dohrenwend, 1984). All these factors contribute to the stresses experienced by women with schizophrenia, in addition to those they face in the parenting role itself.

Mentally ill parents can become trapped in a vicious cycle – environmental stressors have an impact on parent and child, exacerbating parental symptoms and child behaviour problems, which in turn contribute to difficulties in interaction between parent and child. These added stressors exacerbate symptoms and may lead to hospital admission for the ill parent, which can result in the child being placed in alternative care. This is likely to cause stress to both parent and child, potentially delaying parental recovery and creating attachment and relationship problems for the family. The complex interactions between parenthood and 'patienthood' for this group warrant further investigation. These are 'multi-distressed' families (Wahler & Graves, 1983), exposed to a wide range of stressors that increase the likelihood of family dysfunction.

Workers from many different service sectors – parent aides, family law court, family services officers, mental health workers and hospital staff – identify mothers with schizophrenia as being more frequent users of services. Many also identify this client group as the hardest to work with and feel least competent in working with mentally ill parents and their children. Segregation of services and professional role boundaries contribute to workers' perceptions in this regard.

Several factors may have contributed to a rising awareness of the needs of mothers with schizophrenia. Deinstitutionalization has meant that many people with mental illness who were previously confined to extended-care facilities are now living in the community. Where institutions generally segregated the sexes and discouraged the development of sexual relationships, the opportunity for motherhood was consequently limited. For some, community care has provided the opportunity to experience the same milestones in life, including parenthood, as do the wider community.

How many women with schizophrenia are mothers?

There is a large body of literature examining fertility (the presence or absence of offspring) and fecundity (the number of children) of men and women with psychotic disorders ((Haverkamp et al., 1982). These studies have been conducted in many different nations over several decades and have used varying levels of design rigour. Despite this, the results of such studies are relatively consistent. Men with schizophrenia tend to have a marked reduction in the number of offspring compared to well control men. Women with psychotic disorders also tend to have fewer offspring, but the gap between these women and non-affected women is less pronounced than for men (Jablensky, 1995).

The factors that contribute to the lower number of offspring in women with schizophrenia are complex and involve features of schizophrenia and its resultant disabilities and handicaps; the impact of medications and hospitalization; and societal factors. It is difficult to delineate the individual impact of each of these interrelated factors on the fertility of women with schizophrenia.

Many of the studies that have examined fertility in schizophrenia have attempted to reconcile findings from genetics and epidemiology. There is robust evidence that genetic factors influence susceptibility to psychoses (Mowry et al., 1997). However, the apparently stable incidence of schizophrenia across time in spite of a reduction in fertility and fecundity (i.e. a negative selection bias) is difficult to explain. It has been proposed that non-affected family members have more children than would be predicted in order to 'compensate' for the impact of schizophrenia on general fertility of affected individuals, but studies that have examined this issue have been inconsistent in their findings (Buck et al., 1975; Ushiroyama et al., 1993; Fananas & Bertranpetit, 1995; Bassett et al., 1996).

Motherhood and schizophrenia: determining the scope and nature of the issues

In a recent study undertaken by the authors (Hearle et al., 1999; McGrath et al., 1999), we examined this issue in a group of patients with psychoses who were in contract with two community mental health clinics and an extended-care psychiatric hospital in Queensland, Australia. Data on diagnosis, age-at-first-diagnosis and number and age of offspring were collected. A genogram of the probands' family was drawn that identified sex, age, affected status and the number of offspring for the patients and their siblings.

From the sample of 342 individuals with psychoses, 110 were women. Most of the women had non-affective psychoses (schizophrenia, $n = 75$, atypical psychoses, $n = 13$). Of 1025 siblings identified in the genograms, 90 were reported to have a psychotic disorder. These affected siblings were excluded from the analysis, leaving 935 unaffected siblings for the group comparisons.

We found that 36% of all patients with psychotic disorders were parents. Most women with psychotic disorders were mothers (65 of 110 women: 59%). In the entire sample of patients with psychoses ($n = 342$), parents had significantly fewer years of education than non-parents ($t = -2.48$, df $= 335$, $p = 0.01$). As expected, parents were more likely to be married or divorced compared to non-parents ($\chi^2 = 181.74$, df $= 2$, $p < 0.001$). Of the parents, 11 (9%) had a partner with a serious mental illness. None of the non-parents had mentally ill partners. Parents and non-parents did not differ on the number of admissions to hospital, nor on the duration of such admissions. No differences were found between parents and non-parents on the following categorical variables: non-English-speaking background, self-reported financial difficulties, type of accommodation and satisfaction with accommodation.

As in other studies, there was a marked reduction in fertility in men with non-affective psychoses when compared to their unaffected brothers (mean number of offspring $= 0.45$ vs. 1.56 respectively). Women with non-affective psychoses had fewer offspring than their well sisters, but this difference did not reach statistical significance (mean number of offspring $= 1.55$ vs. 1.91 respectively). A similar picture was found for women with affective psychoses (mean number of offspring $= 1.74$ vs. 1.95); however, the small number of women with affective psychoses ($n = 22$) limits interpretation of the data.

A partial correlation was undertaken in order to examine whether age-at-first-diagnosis was associated with mean number of offspring. A weak but statistically significant relationship emerged, indicating that those with an earlier age-at-first-diagnosis tended to have fewer children ($r = 0.15$, $n = 322$, $p < 0.001$). These data support the notion that the later age of onset for schizophrenia in women may be a contributing factor for the relative increased fertility in women with schizophrenia compared to men with schizophrenia.

In addition to motherhood, we looked at reproductive issues in the sample. The 110 women in the survey had had a total of 257 pregnancies, resulting in 198 live births. A total of 134 (52%) of the pregnancies had been unplanned. Of the unplanned pregnancies, 25% had ended in termination. None of the planned pregnancies had been terminated. Concerning the offspring, 94 (47%) had been born before the mother's diagnosis was made, whilst 71 (36%) were born after the mother's diagnosis was made, and 16 (8%) in the year of initial diagnosis (data missing for 17 offspring). Eighteen (16%) mothers reported that at least one of their psychiatric admissions had been within 6 months of the birth of one of their children.

We also asked the women with both affective and non-affective psychoses about their plans to have children in the future. Five women who were already mothers indicated that they would like to have more children; 12 non-mothers indicated that they would eventually like to have children; and 18 non-mothers indicated that they preferred never to have children. Of those who were postmenopausal, only 4 had not had children.

Examining the parent group, 36 had one offspring, 37 had two offspring, 26 had three offspring, while 25 had four or more offspring (total off-spring = 323). Of the parents, 27 fathers and 21 mothers (14% of all participants) had children under the age of 16 years. Of the parents with children less than 16 years of age, 20 (42%) had their children living with them. In total, there were 75 offspring who were aged under 16 years. Of these, 34 resided with the index patients and 24 with the other parent (often the well parent after separation), whilst a further 4 lived with relatives other than the patient's partner (or former partner) and 5 were in permanent foster care or adoption. The whereabouts of 3 children was unknown to the parent.

Who helps mothers with psychotic disorders care for their children?

Concerning child care, most parents had relied on relatives for assistance ($n = 97$; 87%: percentages exclude missing data), while 24% ($n = 27$) relied on friends. Other forms of child care included: foster care ($n = 15$; 13.5%), crèche ($n = 3$; 4%), day care ($n = 3$; 3%) and emergency respite care ($n = 6$; 5%). Five children had been placed in permanent adoption (4.5%).

Parents were asked whether they had received assistance or interventions specifically related to child care from government and non-government agencies. Nineteen parents (18%) reported interventions from the state-government statutory child protection agency. Parents also reported child-care assistance or interventions organized by the following agencies: mental health clinics ($n = 14$; 13%), church groups ($n = 11$; 10%), psychiatric hospitals ($n = 9$; 8%), general community agencies ($n = 9$; 8%), legal aid services ($n = 6$; 6%), maternity hospitals ($n = 6$; 6%) and family courts ($n = 5$; 5%). Of the parents, 13 (11%) stated that they had received intervention relating to care of their child against their will.

Parents were also asked whether certain prespecified factors had impeded access to ideal child-care assistance. The most frequently endorsed factor was the desire to manage alone ($n = 52$; 49%). Other factors include an inability to pay for help ($n = 42$; 40%), not thought of seeking help ($n = 40$; 37%), not knowing where to get help ($n = 38$; 36%), a fear that children would be removed from the parent ($n = 32$; 30%), being too embarrassed to ask for help ($n = 23$; 22%), no services available in the subject's vicinity ($n = 22$; 21%) and having asked for but not received help ($n = 13$; 12%).

The needs of mothers with schizophrenia

Individuals with schizophrenia have a range of needs related to their core illness and associated disablement. The needs of mothers with schizophrenia have much in common with the needs of other parents; however, there are several particular areas that require attention. Once again, the empirically based literature about the needs of mothers with psychosis is scant.

A recent non-systematic survey of parents with a mental illness ($n = 70$) identified needs such as assistance with explaining mental illness to their children, respite from the children, parent support groups and supportive and practical in-home care (Cowling, 1996). Another study (Wang & Goldschmidt, 1996), based on interviews with mentally ill parents with dependent children ($n = 50$), found that 25% of the families had offspring placed in institutions or foster care. A sizeable subgroup (40%) reported that they had never received professional help related to their children, and a third of the parents expressed a need for support that had not been received. Many of the participants stated that they did not know where to go for help or would not be comfortable doing so. These issues were explored with mentally ill mothers (including 8 with self-reported 'psychotic disorders') and case managers (Nicholson et al., 1998a, b). Key themes to emerge from the focus group discussions included issues related to the stigma of mental illness, the difficulties of dealing with general day-to-day parenting, the impact of managing mental illness and the fear of losing contact with children. There is a paucity of data on the experiences and needs of fathers with mental illness.

How can we improve outcomes for mothers with schizophrenia and their offspring?

Most parents find the demands of the parenting role stressful and challenging at times, as well as enormously satisfying. For mothers with schizophrenia there may be the added stressors of coping with their symptoms and consequent disability, as well as the impact of being a marginalized and stigmatized group in our society. All parents at times become concerned for the future of their children, but for mothers with schizophrenia there is the added burden of fear that their children may also develop a mental illness. This fear is very real, and is reinforced in the research literature that shows an increased risk for the children of parents with serious mental illness (Gottesman & Shields, 1976).

Less is known about the complex interactions of genetic risk and environmental influences. Other family-related factors which pose a risk to the psychological and social development of children are commonly found in families where a parent has mental illness. Low socioeconomic status (Jellinek et al, 1991), limited parental social skills and social support (Goldstein, 1987; Liberman, 1982), negative affect of the parent (Laroche et al., 1987), overcrowded living conditions (Rutter & Quinton, 1974) and impaired functioning in marital roles (Webster, 1990; Patterson et al., 1997) may all exert a significant effect on a child's development. The severity and chronicity of parental mental illness, the frequency and duration of separations due to hospital admissions and characteristics of the children themselves are all factors influencing outcome for the children.

Both the health and family services systems have often largely ignored the particular issues faced by mothers with schizophrenia. Services have been developed to meet the needs of the particular organization, or to utilize the skills of their staff, rather than to meet the complex needs of their client group. Health services tend to focus on the treatment of symptoms of individual clients, whilst family services concentrate on assessing of parental competence or child protection. This has led to compartmentalized services that exclude clients who are not seen to be those organizations' constituents; this has erected barriers to easy access to such services. The increasing competition for the welfare dollar is likely to mean that this tendency to exclude clients by considering them to belong to another services' area of responsibility will increase.

As discussed above, the interaction between motherhood and mental illness is a complex one, and involves many factors. For many mentally ill parents there is a need to access multiple services – legal, family, health (physical and mental), housing and financial, to name but a few. Negotiating the complicated web of services to achieve the desired outcome is a difficult task for anyone. For those with problems such as poor cognitive skills and difficulty in concentration, or for those experiencing symptoms such as hallucinations or delusions, the task is even more arduous. The following case scenarios highlight some of these issues.

Case vignette 1:

Patricia developed schizophrenia in her late teenage years. In her mid-20s she became pregnant and acutely psychotic following the birth of her son. Whilst acutely unwell, she expressed delusions about her baby to obstetric staff. Concerned about the baby, staff contacted child protection services who took court action to gain guardianship of the child. Eventually Patricia made a good response to medication, and was no longer considered to be a threat to her child. Issues of loss and grief were prominent for Patricia. A 3-year legal battle ensued between mother, grandmother and the child protection agency – expensive for all in both monetary and emotional terms. Mental health and child protection professionals had opposing views arising from conflicting priorities and differing background knowledge and expertise. The clients (mother, grandmother or baby, depending on which service was involved) lacked trust in any service or professional, and felt let down by all – a situation encouraged by their legal counsel who advised them to talk to no one. Guardianship of the child was eventually granted to the grandmother, who then faced the difficult situation of removing her grandson from his foster mother who had cared for the child for 3 years. The emotional trauma to all concerned is beyond measure – the poor outcome for all after an enormous input of resources is of great concern.

This case is far from isolated. Consumers of mental health services who are parents tell movingly of the difficulties they have faced in parenting their children. Of concern to service providers in particular is the reluctance of many consumers to seek help for fear of losing custody of their children. This remains a valid fear, as parental psychiatric illness has been shown to be not only a common contributing factor for children being taken into care, but also for those children remaining in care for protracted periods (Isaac et al., 1986).

Case vignette 2:

> Bill and May both suffer from schizophrenia. They have a 17-year-old daughter with whom they are barely acquainted. Child protection workers, responding to concerns of neglect, removed her from their care as an infant and placed her with a foster family. She was sexually abused within the foster family and moved on to another family-based programme. Later she was moved to a teenage girls' hostel where she rein-stigated contact with her parents. Both parents and child feel enormous anger towards the service systems which they blame for having denied them a relationship, and for having failed to provide a secure and loving home for the child. Again, the systems in place to assist this family were inadequate, and the experiences for all concerned were damaging.

What is it about services for mothers with schizophrenia that is so wrong? Although sharing a common client group, it is rare for different service sectors to consult with each other. It is more common for them to find fault with each other and blame others for poor client outcomes. They rarely share a common focus of intervention or knowledge base and often have conflicting aims. For example, mental health services focus on the treatment of the parent's illness primarily and may also consider how best to support the parent and improve her quality of life. Although taking a more holistic approach in more recent years, they are often regarded as constrained by a traditional medical model. Family services are often divided into different streams – child protection, juvenile justice, alternative care – and are primarily interested in the child and how to promote the best outcomes as they see it, for the child. Legal services advocate on behalf of their client, regardless of the welfare of others involved, and function according to legal precedent.

These services, as well as others such as general practitioners, education and child care, may all be engaged with a family at the same time, leading to further confusion for the mother. Thus, a mother may be inundated with workers who often give conflicting advice and make multiple demands. The mother may not identify a need for any of these services. Mental health workers may be encouraging their clients to continue in a parenting role, seeing it as good motivation for the parent to comply with treatment and perform well for the sake of the child. Concurrently a child welfare worker may be encouraging the parent to relinquish custodial care, seeing this as the best outcome for the child. Mothers with schizophrenia who do not manage this 'systems abuse' can unwittingly reinforce professionals' views that they are too sick to parent their children.

Social services agencies may become involved, perhaps to assist with placement or because of concerns of abuse or neglect of a child by a stressed mother with schizophrenia. Many psychiatrically disabled parents (in common with all parents) have a fear of professional interference. This is understandable for many reasons. Psychiatry has traditionally alienated families by implicating them in causing illnesses in their relatives. Families and patients remember feeling blamed by now discredited theories of the 'schizophrenogenic' mother and the 'double-bind' communication pattern that supposedly caused psychiatric illness in children. Psychiatrically disabled parents may be used to seeing themselves in the familiar patient role, at times treated without their consent and held in hospital against their will by mental health legislation. It is not surprising that many parents with schizophrenia do not ask for help with child care because they fear that their children will be taken away.

In these times of economic rationalization and increased competition for the funding dollar, it is increasingly important to maximize client outcomes and improve the efficiency and effectiveness of our services. As discussed above, not only is our current organization of service delivery and practice often not achieving this, but in many respects it hampers efficient use of resources and minimizes client outcomes. Intersectoral collaboration is a major difficulty in most service environments. Problems can be seen at many levels, from the individual worker, the agency and the service structure, to the lack of clear policy direction and political will to provide sufficient funds for services for mothers with schizophrenia.

As previously noted, mentally ill parents have multiple and complex service needs across a spectrum of sectors. Housing, health (both physical and mental), income security, disability and family support are some of the most widely utilized and all are likely to impose a complicated set of rules and regulations that must be rigorously followed for benefits to be gained. If not, exclusion can be swift and appeal and reinstatement difficult.

In many regions, the reality is that health and social service systems are fragmented. Commonwealth or federal, state and local governments do not always have agreed policies and sometimes have competing agendas. At the service delivery level, there are many services working with mentally ill mothers, often lacking any coordination or understanding of each other's role. Sometimes they may be working with one family member in isolation, or may be a specialist lacking knowledge and expertise in other areas. The impact of parental mental illness often draws support from the extended family; grandparents become major care-givers, while siblings may be carers for each other and at times for their unwell parent. Given that parental mental illness can have detrimental effects on the whole family and is often regarded as a family problem, a family-centred approach to support is necessary.

Combining the knowledge and skills of workers from health and family services should provide for best practice, but often does not. In looking at why this is so, a number of problems can be identified. Different services identify different clients. Mental health services continue to focus on the individual patient and are governed by strict codes of confidentiality. Consumers may understandably be very reluctant for their mental health worker to contact other agencies to coordinate their approach. Child protection services have a statutory role and clearly see the children as their clients, as does the education system. Other services may see the whole family as the client or represent one family member only.

Not only do the services identify different clients, but they tend to target different problems. For health and mental health services, the illness is usually regarded as the problem and thus the treatment of symptoms is generally the major focus. Mental health workers may only see clients at the hospital or clinic and be unaware of problems in the home environment or the situation of dependent children. Child protection or family support workers may consider the problem to be a lack of parenting skills, neglect of the children, poor motivation or disorganized home environment, and may lack an understanding of the impact of the parents' illness on their ability to fulfil their role.

Conclusions

The results of our local study, detailed in this chapter, support the finding that parenthood for the mentally ill can be associated with grief, loss and frustration (Human Rights and Equal Opportunity Commission, 1993). Only a minority of the offspring resided with the index parents (17%), and many parents expressed a desire for more contact with their children and adult offspring. Over 10% of parents reported past interventions against their will related to the care of their children, and nearly a third of parents stated that they were reluctant to access help with child care because they feared that their children would be removed from them.

The study also provides insights into the pattern of child-care utilization in parents with a psychotic disorder. Clearly, the support of family and friends is often relied upon. This finding has implications for those parents who do not have such support, and one could speculate that the social network available to assist mentally ill parents may be a crucial factor in a range of parent, offspring and family-functioning outcome variables. In addition, the child-care role taken on by family and friends in times of need also reminds service providers about the importance of informal care-givers. Provision of timely and practical support related to child care for these individuals, in addition to the index patients, may serve to keep such support networks intact. We agree with other researchers who have commented on the important role that a supportive social support network can play in keeping children within the family system (Wang & Goldschmidt, 1996; Miller, 1997; Nicholson, et al., 1998b). It may be argued that those parents who do not have such social networks are more likely to seek assistance from community agencies in relation to caring for their children.

Many parents with psychoses identified that they needed support, but were unable to access this for various reasons. Many parents experienced financial barriers to accessing optimal child care, while others reported that there were no suitable services in their local area. About 12% of parents reported no response following requests for help with child care. Service providers should be able to address these factors. Other factors that impeded access to optimal child care (e.g. embarrassment, fear of loss of child) require consumer education and practical demonstrations that services respect the needs of parents with psychotic illnesses. Consumer involvement in service development may assist in building trust between parents and service providers.

Whilst this chapter has concentrated on the needs of mothers with schizophrenia who have contact with their children, it is also important to note that many childless patients with psychoses reported a desire for future parenthood. Practical education about the responsibilities of parenthood need to be incorporated into family planning – a point that has been made repeatedly (Bachrach, 1984; Mowbray et al., 1997). In our desire to improve services for parents with mental illness, it is important that we do not neglect the needs of parents with psychotic illness who may have lost their children for various reasons (e.g. being unable to be custodial parents). For those who have lost all contact with their offspring, the impact of this loss on their mental state and their feelings of self-efficacy needs to be recognized.

Currently, there is no framework for provision of services to the family unit, but rather the focus is on the adults and their mental health problem or the children and their care and protection needs. Service philosophies that focus on the functioning and maintenance of the family unit are vital in maintaining intact families and promoting positive outcomes for both parents and children (Nicholson et al., 1993; White et al., 1995; Cohler et al., 1996; Seeman, 1996; Miller, 1997). These services need to be evaluated from a range of perspectives.

Finally, we speculate that the economic costs of providing timely assistance to these families and their immediate support networks may be substantially lower than the cost of services that may subsequently be required from government agencies if these families do not remain intact. Apart from the psychological costs to the parents and offspring, more long-term research is required to estimate the costs of *not* providing optimal care to parents with schizophrenia (Rupp & Keith, 1993).

REFERENCES

Bachrach, L.L. (1984). Deinstitutionalization and women: assessing the consequences of public policy. *Am. Psychol.* **39**, 1171–7.

Bassett, A.S., Bury, A., Hodgkinson, K.A. & Honer, W.G. (1996). Reproductive fitness in familial schizophrenia. *Schizophr. Res.*, **21**, 151–60.

Buck, C., Hobbs, G.E., Simpson, H. & Wanklin, J.M. (1975). Fertility of the sibs of schizophrenic patients. *Br. J. Psychiatry*, **127**, 235–9.

Cohler, B.J., Stott, F.M. & Musick, J.S. (1996). Distressed parents and their young children: interventions for families at risk. In *Parental Psychiatric Disorders: Distressed Parents and their Families*, 1st edn, ed. M. Göpfert, J. Webster & M.V. Seeman, pp. 107–34. Cambridge: Cambridge University Press.

Cowling, V. (1996). Meeting the support needs of families with dependent children where a parent has a mental illness. *Fam. Matters*, **45**, 22–5.

Dohrenwend, B.S. & Dohrenwend, B.P. (1984). *Stressful Life Events: Their Nature and Effect*. New York: Wiley.

Fananas, L. & Bertranpetit, J. (1995). Reproductive rates in families of schizophrenic patients in a case-control study. *Acta Psychiatr. Scand.*, **91**, 202–4.

Goldstein, S. (1987). Bye bye Brady Bunch. *Family Ther. Networker*, **10**, 31–2.

Goodman, S.H. (1984). Children of disturbed parents: the interface between research and intervention. *Am. J. Commun. Psychol.*, **12**, 663–87.

Gottesman, I.I. & Shields, J. (1976). Rejoinder toward optimal arousal and away from original sin. *Schizophr. Bull.*, **2**, 447–53

Haverkamp, F., Propping, P. & Hilger, T. (1982). Is there an increase of reproductive rates in schizophrenics? I. Critical review of the literature. *Arch. Psychiatr. Nervenkr.*, **232**, 439–50.

Hearle J., Plant, K., Jenner, L., Barkla, J. & McGrath, J.J. (1999). A survey of contact with offspring and assistance with child care among parents with psychotic disorders. *Psychiatr. Serv.*, **50**, 1354–6.

Human Rights and Equal Opportunity Commission (1993). *Human Rights and Mental Illness*. Canberra: Australian Government Publishing Service.

Isaac, B.C., Minty, E.B. & Morrison, R.M. (1986). Children in care: the association with mental disorder in the parents. *Br. J. Soc. Work*, **16**, 325–9.

Jablensky, A. (1995). Schizophrenia: the epidemiological horizon. In *Schizophrenia*, ed. S.R. Hirsch and D.R. Weinberger, pp. 206–52. Oxford: Blackwell Science.

Jellinek, M.S., Bishop, S.S., Murphy, J.M., Biederman, J. & Rosenbaum, J. (1991). Screening for dysfunction in the children of outpatients at a psychopharmacology unit. *Am. J. Psychiatry*, **148**, 1031–6.

Laroche, C., Sheiner, R., Lester, E. et al. (1987). Children of parents with manic-depressive illness: a follow-up study. *Can. J. Psychiatry*, **32**, 563–9.

Liberman, R.P. (1982). Assessment of social skills *Schizophr. Bull.*, **8**, 62–83.

McGrath, J.J., Hearle, J., Jenner, L., Plant, K., Drummond, A. & Barkla, J.M. (1999). The fertility and fecundity of patients with psychoses. *Acta Psychiatr. Scand.*, **99**, 441–6.

Miller, L.J. (1997). Sexuality, reproduction, and family planning in women with schizophrenia. *Schizophr. Bull.*, **23**, 623–35.

Mowbray, C.T., Oyserman, D. & Ross, B.A. (1997). Parenting and the significance of women with serious mental illness. *Am. J. Orthopsychiatry*, **65**, 21–38.

Mowry, B., Nancarrow, D. & Levinson, D. (1997). The molecular genetics of schizophrenia: an update. *Aust. N.Z. J. Psychiatry*, **31**, 704–13.

Nicholson, J., Geller, J., Fisher, W. &. Dion, G.L. (1993). State policies and programs that address the needs of mentally ill mothers in the public sector. *Hosp. Commun. Psychiatry*, **44**, 484–9.

Nicholson, J., Sweeny, E.M. & Geller, J. (1998a). Mothers with mental illness: I. The competing demands of parenting and living with mental illness. *Psychiatr. Serv.*, **49**, 635–42.

Nicholson, J., Sweeny, E.M. & Geller, J. (1998b). Mothers with mental illness: II. Family relationships and the context of parenting. *Psychiatr. Serv.*, **49**, 643–49.

Oates, M. (1997). Patients as parents: the risk to children. *Br. J. Psychiatry*, **170**, 22–7.

Patterson, T.L., Semple, S.J., Shaw, W.S. et al. (1997). Self-reported social functioning among older patients with schizophrenia. *Schizophr. Res.,* **27**, 199–210.

Rupp, A. & Keith, S.J. (1993). The costs of schizophrenia: assessing the burden. *Psychiatr. Clin. North Am.*, **16**, 413–23.

Rutter, J.E. & Quinton, D. (1984). Parental psychiatric disorder: effects on children. *Psychol. Med.*, **14**, 853–880.

Sand, S. (1995). The parenting experience of low-income single women with serious mental disorders. *Fam. Soc. J. Contemp. Hum. Serv.*, **2**, 86–96.

Schwab, B., Clark, R. & Drake, R. (1991). An ethnographic note on clients as parents. *Psychosoc. Rehab. J.*, **15**, 95–9.

Seeman, M.V. (1996). The mother with schizophrenia. In *Parental Psychiatric Disorder*, ed. M. Göpfert, M.V. Seeman and J. Webster, 1st edn., pp. 190–200. Cambridge: Cambridge University Press.

Ushiroyama, T., Tsubokura, S., Okamoto, Y. & Sugimoto, O. (1993). [Clinical study of pregnant women with psychotic disorders during last 14 years in Osaka Medical College]. *Nippon Sanka Fujinka Gakkai Zasshi*, **45**, 347–54.

Wahler, R.G. & Graves, M. (1983). Setting events in social networks: ally or enemy in child behavior therapy. *Behav. Ther.*, **14**, 19–36.

Wang, A. & Goldschmidt, V. (1996). Interviews with psychiatric inpatients about professional intervention with regard to their children. *Acta Psychiatr. Scand.*, **93**, 57–61.

Webster, C. (1990). Stress: a potential disruptor of parent perceptions and family interactions. *J. Clin. Child Psychol.*, **19**, 302–12.

White, C., Nicholson, J., Fisher, W. & Geller, J. (1995). Mothers with severe mental illness caring for children. *J. Nerv. Ment. Dis.*, **183**, 398–403.

8

Women and schizophrenia: treatment implications

Paul Fitzgerald and Mary V. Seeman

The data presented in this book on sex differences in schizophrenia can inform prevention and treatment strategies. In particular, we concern ourselves here with those prevention and treatment issues which have particular relevance for women with schizophrenia. The reader is also referred to Chapter 5 for a more detailed consideration of hormonal aspects of schizophrenia in women, and treatment implications thereof.

There are a number of avenues for the prevention of illness in subsequent generations that apply particularly to women. These include sex education and counselling, prevention of sexual victimization, the prevention of the transmission of sexual diseases and of unwanted pregnancy, prenatal programming and safeguards against obstetric complications. Prophylactic help with parenting is of paramount importance and is likely to play an important role in the amelioration or prevention of a range of psychiatric disorders. For a more detailed consideration of these issues, the reader is referred to Chapters 6 and 7.

With respect to treatment, men and women have somewhat different needs. The particular needs of women include paying attention to pregnancy status, parental status, menstrual status, concurrent use of oral contraceptives or replacement hormones and thyroid status. Older women may need to be screened for osteoporosis and bladder insufficiency prior to the prescription of neuroleptics. In both sexes, the lean/fat weight ratio is important, as is muscle activity for those on depot medications. Medical and chronic pain history may reveal the use of concomitant medications which interact with prescribed drugs. Alcohol and drug use (including tea, coffee and smoking) is of special relevance.

Sexuality

Due to the confounding variable of institutionalization, early studies exploring the sexuality of patients with schizophrenia appear to have underestimated the degree of normal sexual activity amongst this group. A number of studies in the 1980s and 1990s, however, have focused on community samples and appear to give a more accurate picture of the sexual lives of patients with schizophrenia. These studies indicate that schizophrenia does not directly limit the sexual interest or desire of female patients, and most are sexually active (Raboch, 1984; Miller, 1997). This is despite the fact that side-effects of antipsychotic medication, including sedation and the gynaecological effects of raised prolactin, may impact negatively on sexual desire and behaviour. Hyperprolactinaemia in particular may result in orgasmic dysfunction and impaired libido.

Of additional concern are the particulars of the sexual lives experienced by women with schizophrenia. Even when socioeconomic effects are accounted for, patients experience higher rates of sexual abuse, feeling pressured to have sex, sex-exchange behaviour and activities that place them at substantial risk for sexually transmitted diseases. These activities include having sex more frequently with homosexual and bisexual partners and having more lifetime partners (Miller & Finnerty, 1996; Coverdale et al., 1997; Miller, 1997). These problems are likely to be multidetermined. Poor judgement, problems with impulse control and high rates of substance abuse may contribute (McCullough et al., 1992). The relative passivity and isolation that accompany schizophrenia may also permit sexual victimization.

Amenorrhoea and menstrual cycle disruption are commonly caused by neuroleptics and this is usually secondary to a rise in prolactin, which may (but not always) prevent ovulation. Pregnancy can, however, occur in the presence of amenorrhoea and may pass unnoticed for several months. Importantly, many of the newer atypical antipsychotics cause less pronounced prolactin rises, and women taking these medications are more likely to become pregnant than those on the more typical antipsychotic agents. Clozapine, quetiapine and olanzapine in particular, are associated with a reduced incidence of prolactin elevation. Women who are changed to these medications following treatment with traditional agents should be advised that the chance of becoming pregnant may increase substantially.

It is important that women with psychotic disorders be counselled about effective contraception, and that clinicians be aware of the risk of pregnancy. Somatic symptoms such as nausea or breast swelling may be prematurely discounted when reported by psychotic women; they may too quickly be attributed to the effects of neuroleptics or related to the psychotic disorder.

When pregnancy is desired, it should be carefully planned taking into consideration the woman's stage of illness, social supports and the likelihood that she will relapse with a withdrawal of medication. It may be appropriate to withdraw neuroleptic therapy before conception, although the evidence for risks associated with antipsychotic medication (other than phenothiazines and butyrophenones) is limited (Altshuler et al., 1996). There is some support for the notion that it may impose less risk for the mother to be continued on low-dose maintenance treatment rather than risk relapse and the possible subsequent exposure to higher doses of medication (Altshuler et al., 1996).

Delivery and the postpartum period

Women on antipsychotic medication should try to taper their medication about 2 weeks prior to anticipated delivery in order to prevent ill effects in the newborn. However, medication should be recommended immediately after the birth to avoid relapse of psychosis in what is a vulnerable period, both in terms of hormonal flux (see Chapter 5), as well as the stresses inherent in having a young child to care for.

Antipsychotic medications taken whilst breast-feeding have not been associated with harm to the infant. However, the experience with the newer antipsychotic medications is necessarily limited, and due caution should be exercised.

Mothers with schizophrenia should be afforded the opportunity to remain in hospital until they feel comfortable with their babies, and home help has been organized. Outpatient care for the first 3–6 months should, where feasible, be arranged in the home, as it may be difficult for these women to attend clinics. Medications must be monitored carefully to ensure adequate dosage, and side-effects need to be checked. Mothers require sensitive guidance and monitoring with respect to feeding, changing nappies and play. The importance of sleep, and the potential for psychotic relapse when sleep patterns go awry, should be borne in mind and problems dealt with promptly.

As soon as possible, mothers should be encouraged to meet other mothers with babies of the same age to form a mutual-aid network. Parents and grandparents may need to be actively recruited to help with baby-sitting. Ongoing education about psychosis, as well as about parenting, should be provided; books and videos can be invaluable.

As soon as feasible after the birth, mothers with schizophrenia should be encouraged to return to rehabilitation programmes and special help should be given in the area of living skills (e.g. budgeting, shopping, cooking). Special attention should be paid to the monitoring of the parenting itself, and acknowledgement made that the parenting role changes with the age of the child. Particular times of stress, for example starting school, should be anticipated and prepared for. Issues relating to women with schizophrenia as parents are further detailed in Chapter 7.

Menopause

The life phase associated with menopause is an important one for patients suffering from, or at risk for developing, psychotic disorders. First, women are at particular risk of developing a new psychotic disorder at this time (see also Chapters 4 and 5). Second, a number of significant psychosocial stressors may emerge during this period, including the death of previously supportive parents, ill health of the patient or spouse, and the departure of children from the home. Third, menopause may play an important role in mediating the course of schizophrenia. Research to date indicates that the severity of schizophrenia levels off in men after their 40s. This may be related to the depletion of dopamine receptors with age – a decline that is more precipitous in men than in women (Wong et al., 1984; see Chapter 2). In women, the loss of the protective effect of estrogen at this time, may serve to exacerbate symptoms (see Chapter 5).

Finally, after menopause all women are at increased risk of developing a variety of medical disorders including osteoporosis and cardiovascular disease. Women treated for a number of premenopausal years with typical neuroleptics are likely to have experienced periods of low circulating estrogen levels relating to menstrual-cycle disturbance secondary to increased prolactin. Periods of low circulating estrogen will contribute to a lowering of bone density and increased risk of atherosclerotic cardiovascular disease. It is probable that these risks will compound the risks associated with normal physiological changes after menopause. It is crucial that these women should be carefully assessed at the time of menopause for hormone replacement therapy. Bone densiometry should specifically be considered to evaluate the degree of bone loss and appropriate therapy instituted. Cardiovascular risk factors should be assessed carefully and appropriate action taken. The markedly high rates of smoking in all patients with schizophrenia will add to their risk for both osteoporosis and cardiovascular disease.

Relationship with the treating clinician

It is increasingly recognized that the therapeutic relationships formed by patients with schizophrenia play an important role in the recovery process, and that a capacity to engage with clinicians may change with the evolution of the individual's illness. Schizophrenia, and in particular negative symptoms, affects the capacity of patients to form and maintain interpersonal relationships that may buffer stressful life experiences. Female patients, who often have intact social skills, are better able to form therapeutic relationships but may be very sensitive to frequent alterations in health-care providers, a situation that regularly occurs in public mental health services.

Traditionally, help for families of patients with schizophrenia has referred to the family of origin, for example counselling offered to the parents and the young adult suffering from schizophrenia. This configuration is more appropriate to the provision of care to males with schizophrenia and their families than to females. Family intervention for women with schizophrenia may, in contrast, mean including partners and/or children. Specific interventions should be developed and applied to the unique difficulties experienced by the children of mothers with schizophrenia. Parents may also be involved in a different role, as potential care-givers for the offspring of women with schizophrenia who are unable to care for their children alone.

Adverse treatment effects

The incidence and severity of various neuroleptic side-effects are confounded by many variables, and heavily dependent on prescribed dose. However, in general it is reasonable to say that, taken together, women experience more adverse neuroleptic side-effects than men do. These include parkinsonism, tardive dyskinesia, agranulocytosis secondary to clozapine and various effects secondary to raised prolactin levels (decreased libido, gynaecomastia, galactorrhoea, amenorrhoea and the secondary effects of estrogen loss, notably osteoporosis and cardiovascular damage). The vulnerability of women to adverse effects is due to higher concentrations of free drug reaching target sites; an enhancement of dopamine blockade by estrogen; a longer duration of storage of neuroleptics in adipose tissue; a higher prevalence of immune reactions in women than in men; and a greater risk in women of drug–drug interactions because of their relatively greater likelihood of comorbid illness (Seeman, 1994).

A clinically relevant point is that the various side-effects of neuroleptics may be of different significance to men and women. As a gross generalization, men are most disturbed by side-effects that interfere with performance, especially sexual performance; women tend to be more disturbed by side-effects which affect appearance – weight gain is especially important (Seeman, 1983).

Extrapyramidal motor side-effects are amongst the more common and disabling side-effects of the older neuroleptics. Acute dystonia, long thought to be more prevalent among men, has been shown in a first-episode fixed-dose 10-week study to occur more readily in women (Casey, 1991). As this author points out, earlier clinical studies did not take into account the fact that young male patients were commonly prescribed higher doses than women, probably because they were perceived as more threatening and their behaviour was seen as requiring higher and more rapid dosing.

A large number of studies have indicated that tardive dyskinesia is more common in female than male patients treated with neuroleptics (Yassa & Jeste, 1992). A more recent cohort (as distinct from a cross-sectional) study, however, found tardive dyskinesia to be more common in elderly men, although its severity was greater in women in their later years (Morgenstern & Glazer, 1993). There is also evidence that the severity and incidence of tardive dyskinesia peak in men at age 50–70, but in women they continue to increase with age (Yassa & Jeste, 1992). It is possible that this pattern and the severity of tardive dyskinesia in elderly women relate to the withdrawal of estrogens at menopause. A number of other explanations have also been offered. One is based upon the observation that tardive dyskinesia may develop more quickly and be more severe when neuroleptics are commenced for the first time later in life, as is more commonly the case in women (Jeste et al., 1992). Another consideration, outlined in Chapter 2, is that the differentially slower rate of loss of dopamine D_2 receptors in females, resulting in a relative excess in late life, compared with men, plays some role in the elevated risk of severe tardive dyskinesia in older women.

As already mentioned, sexual side-effects are commonly experienced by women taking antipsychotic medication. Symptoms may include galactorrhoea, breast engorgement, decreased libido, orgasmic dysfunction and difficulties with lubrication and arousal. This is a crucial area of enquiry as these symptoms are not usually revealed spontaneously by patients and may lead to unacknowledged non-compliance.

Weight gain is a side-effect that may be particularly important in women due to social concerns of body image as well as to its contribution as a cardiovascular risk factor. Weight gain may occur with all neuroleptics but appears to be particularly common with some atypical antipsychotics, possibly due to blockade of histamine or serotonin receptors. Patients need to be carefully monitored and advised in advance as to the benefits of increased physical activity and appropriate dietary alterations.

Another concern with antipsychotic medication relates to the impact that it may have on a mother's capacity to provide adequate supervision and responsiveness during parenting. Clinicians frequently warn of concerns with sedating or hypotensive effects of drugs with respect to driving and operating machinery, but the safety of dependants is often overlooked. This danger is exacerbated by the frequent concomitant use of antidepressants in women with schizophrenia. All antidepressants can be combined with neuroleptics at their usual effective dose but side-effects common to both, such as sedation and hypotension, are additive, so dose increments must be prescribed more gradually than usual. The use of serotonin reuptake inhibitors may increase the plasma level of neuroleptics and, therefore, more adverse (as well as beneficial) effects may result. There have also been reports of confusional episodes resulting from a combination of lithium and neuroleptics and their concomitant use has been suggested as a potential risk factor for neuroleptic malignant syndrome.

Hormonal therapy

As has been addressed in Chapters 4 and 5, it is crucial to consider the hormonal status of any woman who is receiving treatment for schizophrenia. Issues that should be addressed in clinical assessment include the history of menstrual functioning, the effect of antipsychotic medication on the menstrual cycle, the use of contraception and planning for pregnancy. It is also important to consider the role of hormonal therapies at various stages in the life cycle of a woman with psychosis.

First, it is crucial to treat women with medication such as to minimize prolactin elevation and preserve normal menstrual cycle function. This requires careful dose titration and the consideration of those atypical antipsychotics that minimally elevate prolactin.

Second, we can consider the role estrogen itself may play as a therapeutic agent (Table 8.1). As has been discussed elsewhere in this book (see Chapter 5), estrogen appears to play an important modulating role in the expression of schizophrenia in a variety of ways. In particular, it acts to modulate dopamine neurotransmission and acts as an antagonist at the dopamine receptor. Its role as a dopamine antagonist raises the possibility of its therapeutic use in psychotic patients in a variety of ways.

No blinded controlled trials of the use of estrogen have been published to date, although a number of case reports and an open clinical trial have indicated that there may be benefits of adding estrogen to standard antipsychotic medication (Dennerstein et al., 1983; Kulkarni et al., 1996). In the study of Kulkarni and colleagues, 11 women treated with antipsychotic medication and estradiol experienced a more rapid response of their psychotic symptoms as compared to the control group. Interestingly, the differences were not sustained by week 8 of the study, indicating that the effect of estrogen was temporary or catalytic, allowing the antipsychotic medication to achieve its maximum effect in a shorter period of time.

At this stage, there is insufficient evidence to argue for the routine use of estrogen as an adjunct to antipsychotic therapy. However, it is import-

Table 8.1. Possible roles of hormonal therapies in female patients with schizophrenia

As adjuvant dopamine antagonist therapy
To ameliorate cyclical symptomatic fluctuation
To preserve bone density and prevent cardiovascular disease
To preserve, enhance or restore fertility
As contraception
As therapy for tardive dyskinesia

ant to ensure that women have the benefits of a normal circulating level of estrogen, and this may require supplementation where there are abnormalities that will not respond to interventions such as adjusting the dose of antipsychotic medication. Additionally, it is reasonable to consider a therapeutic trial of estrogen where the patient experiences an exacerbation of symptoms that clearly appear to relate to fluctuating hormonal levels through the menstrual cycle, or in women with resistant symptoms. Other phases in life where estrogen levels are low may also be appropriate times for hormonal interventions. The benefits of hormone replacement therapy at the time of menopause for bone density and cardiovascular status have already been addressed, but it may also prove to be the case that postmenopausal estrogen therapy may directly benefit psychotic symptoms.

Conversely, and at this stage theoretically, cyclical variations in circulating estrogen levels may also influence the clinical requirement for antipsychotic medication. There is evidence that psychotic symptoms worsen in low-estrogen phases of the menstrual cycle (Hallonquist et al., 1993; Gattaz et al., 1994; Riecher-Rössler et al., 1994). This raises the possibility that it may be therapeutically appropriate to vary the dose of antipsychotic medication during the menstrual cycle with proportionally higher doses taken in the second half of the cycle when estrogen levels fall. In the maintenance phase of the treatment cycle, this may allow the overall dose of medication administered to be lower, with possible reductions in side-effects, including tardive dyskinesia.

Finally, there may also be a role for estrogen in the treatment of tardive dyskinesia. A number of small open studies have demonstrated some benefit although these have been of a limited magnitude (Villeneuve et al., 1980; Koller et al., 1982; Glazer et al., 1984).

Implications for neuroleptic drug trials

Women have been underrepresented in trials of neuroleptic medication and this has had a significant impact upon our ability to interpret the results of these trials in making decisions about appropriate therapy for female patients. The response of men and women to psychotropic medication varies in a number of important pharmacokinetic and pharmacodynamic ways. These differences influence the individual response to medications, the incidence and type of side-effects experienced and interactions with other medication. Issues of differential expression of schizophrenia in men and women highlight the importance of including women in efficacy trials of antipsychotic drugs. As mentioned, different dosing schedules may be required and, in women, there may be exacerbating or ameliorating effects of menstrual phase, pregnancy, postpartum period, perimenopause and postmenopause. It is therefore important not only to include women but also to include them at various reproductive life stages. Hormonal factors influence bioavailability of drugs at target sites. In addition, sexually dimorphic features, such as the distribution and extent of adipose tissue, vary at different ages and may result in shorter or longer drug half-lives. This influences decisions regarding wash-out and cross-over times, and determines withdrawal effects, cumulative effects and maintenance effects after drug discontinuation (Yonkers et al., 1992). These issues need to be carefully addressed in the development and prescription of new therapies.

There are also broader issues that we must consider when looking at the lack of participation of women in medication trials. For example, we should consider whether women are as likely to enter trials from an adequate position of informed consent. It has been suggested that they are more prone 'to go along' for fear of offending their care-givers and because they have no sense of control over their care (Sherwin, 1992). Women may feel uncomfortable with the non-egalitarian nature of the clinical researcher/ clinical trial subject dyad but favour equal representation for the sake of their political conscience, thus being torn between unacceptable options

(Sherwin, 1992). Women as health consumers may insist on more feminine input into research questions and research protocols. This might include more naturalistic observations and the inclusion of more qualitative measures.

Pharmacokinetic issues

Men and women differ in the ways in which their bodies respond to medication. They have different rates of gastrointestinal drug absorption, different extents of sequestration into adipose tissue, different rates of distribution in the body, different enzymatic activity and liver clearance. A major difference in the kinetics of drug metabolism results from the greater adipose content of female bodies and this difference is especially enhanced with age. As most psychotropic drugs are lipophilic, they are more widely distributed in women, resulting in a longer duration of action. This may result in less rebound and withdrawal phenomena after drug discontinuation but proportionally more danger of toxicity and the requirement for longer wash-out periods. Time of the month (Endicott & Halbreich, 1988; Palmer et al., 1991), weight fluctuations, activity levels, smoking, alcohol intake and diet all distinguish male and female subjects and influence drug clearance via both liver and kidney. Additionally, differences in hormonal milieu in the central nervous system will affect the interaction of psychotropic medication at receptor sites, further altering the clinical response to medication (Yonkers et al., 1992). All of these issues are relevant in the prescription of psychotropic medication. Dosing and safety studies need to consider these differences carefully and produce recommendations appropriate to both sexes.

Measurement of response to treatment

As has previously been discussed, women present with differing symptom patterns from men. The response of symptoms in women needs to be carefully considered in trials, rather than making assumptions about the generalizability of responses across the sexes. Psychological tendencies which differentiate the two sexes (e.g. help-seeking, adherence to prescribed drug regimens) also profoundly affect the interpretation of results of clinical change (Mogul, 1985). Interpersonal factors, as between prescriber and patient, are also important. Women who volunteer for drug trials tend to be especially sensitive to issues of significance to women, such as power differentials, and this needs to be appreciated when interpreting results (Sherwin, 1992).

Safety issues in medication trials

Women must be included in safety trials of new psychotropic agents for a number of reasons. First, the toxicity of drugs may be affected by alterations in the female hormonal milieu that occur at various life stages (Hamilton & Parry, 1983; Halbriech, 1994) such as the menopause. These effects may be directly related to drug action or influenced by factors such as weight fluctuations.

Second, women and men vary in the incidence and type of medical comorbid illnesses. For instance, the extent of alcohol use and smoking varies substantially between the sexes (Haring et al., 1989). Extensive drug and alcohol abuse (not smoking) is usually an exclusion criterion in drug trials but needs to be taken into account when prescribing. Women are also more likely than men to be taking specific concomitant medications, such as anti-inflammatory drugs or sedatives, which affect the plasma levels of psychotropic medication (Ashton, 1991). While significant medical and neurological disease is an exclusion criterion in most drug trials, more minor complaints which necessitate analgesic and other drug use (fibromyalgia, irritable bowel syndrome, insomnia, chronic fatigue, osteoarthritis, hot flushes, nausea) may not exclude the subject (more often than not a woman) but may lead to potential misinterpretation of study results.

Third, there are a number of specific issues to consider. Sexual side-effects are frequently not reported in clinical trials and they need to be specifically elicited, as women often do not report them spontaneously. Medications may also increase the risk of gynaecological or breast malignancy or other illnesses that will rarely arise in male subjects. Special concerns of elderly women also need to be safeguarded. These include drug effects which lead to hypotension, falls and potential broken hips (Ray et al., 1989; Preskorn, 1993).

Fourth, it is vital to consider the effects of prescribed medications on the offspring – born or as yet unborn – of a treated woman. Pregnant women, or those who may fall pregnant, are systematically excluded from trials of new medication. These trials usually require women of child-bearing age to have a negative pregnancy test and to be following a reliable method of contraception prior to entry into a study. Such precautions are understandable but, once the drug is on the market, it may be prescribed, unknowingly, to potentially pregnant women while its effects on the vulnerable developing nervous system of the human fetus remain largely unknown. For example, there is little known about the effects of a number of the newer atypical antipsychotic medications such as risperidone, olanzapine and quetiapine on the developing fetus.

There is no easy answer to this difficulty, as the recruitment of pregnant women into trials of new medications is as problematic as their exclusion. What is necessary is that this issue be addressed seriously by academics and the pharmaceutical industry and that novel solutions be generated. Clinicians will continue to face the difficulty of prescribing for pregnant women and are currently guided only by defensively worded statements to the effect that using certain medications will have uncertain results and cannot be recommended. Programmes of systematic collection of post-marketing data regarding drugs used in pregnancy are required, and clinicians need to be encouraged to report this use without the fear of sanctions and litigation for not having followed restrictive prescribing guidelines.

In considering the welfare of the offspring of women in clinical trials we need to look beyond issues of pregnancy and lactation. Women are usually the care-givers (of children, parents, the ill and disabled) and drug effects during trials will have an impact on those they look after. Subjects in clinical trials are warned not to drive when first starting a new drug but no assurance is requested that mothers of young children have a co-care-taker available when they are first being started on a new medication which may cause dizziness, forgetfulness or sedation. The effect of maternal medication consumption on children has not been systematically addressed in research and this remains an ignored outcome measure in clinical trials.

Conclusions

In this chapter we have considered a variety of clinically relevant issues for the treatment of women with schizophrenia. They differ in a variety of ways from the treatments required in men. There needs to be an expanded focus in clinical treatment and research on issues pertaining to the sexuality of women with schizophrenia, pregnancy and the postpartum period, complications that emerge with menopause, drug dosing and differential rates of side-effects and the role of various hormonal therapies in women with schizophrenia. It is important to note that evidence based upon studies of predominantly male subjects may not be at all applicable to outcome in women.

REFERENCES

Altshuler, L., Cohen, L., Szuba, M. et al. (1996). Pharmacologic management of psychiatric illness during pregnancy: dilemmas and guidelines. *Am. J. Psychiatry*, **153**, 592–606.

Ashton, H. (1991). Psychotropic drug prescribing for women. *Br. J. Psychiatry*, **158** (Suppl. 10), 30–5.

Casey, D. (1991). Neuroleptic drug-induced extrapyramidal syndromes and tardive dyskinesia. *Schizophr. Res.*, **4**, 109–20.

Coverdale, J., Turbott, S. & Roberts, H. (1997). Family planning needs and STD risk behaviours of female psychiatric out-patients. *Br. J. Psychiatry*, **171**, 69–72.

Dennerstein, L., Judd, F. & Davies, B. (1983). Psychosis and the menstrual cycle. *Med. J. Aust.*, **1**, 524–6.

Endicott, J. & Halbreich, U. (1988). Clinical significance of premenstrual dysphoric changes. *J. Clin. Psychiatry*, **49**, 486–9.

Gattaz, W., Vogel, P., Riecher-Rössler, A. et al. (1994). Influence of the menstrual cycle phase on the therapeutic response in schizophrenia. *Biol. Psychiatry*, **36**, 137–9.

Glazer, W., Naftolin, F., Morgenstern, H. et al. (1984). Estrogen replacement and tardive dyskinesia. *Psychoneuroendocrinology*, **10**, 345–50.

Halbreich, U. (1994). Gender-related biological research: methodological and ethical considerations (abstract). *Neuropsychopharmacology*, **10**, 7945.

Hallonquist, J., Seeman, M.V., Lang, M. et al. (1993). Variation in symptom severity over the menstrual cycle of schizophrenics. *Biol. Psychiatry*, **33**, 207–9.

Hamilton, J. & Parry, B. (1983). Sex-related differences in clinical drug response: Implications for women's health. *J. Am. Med. Women's Assoc.*, **231**, 375–9.

Haring, C., Meise, U., Humpel, C. et al. (1989). Dose-related plasma levels of clozapine: Influence of smoking behaviour, sex and age. *Psychopharmacology*, **99**, S38–40.

Jeste, D., Kleinman, J., Potkin, S. et al. (1992). Ex uno multi: subtyping the schizophrenia syndrome. *Biol. Psychiatry*, **17**, 199–222.

Koller, W., Barr, A. & Biary, N. (1982). Estrogen treatment of dyskinetic disorders. *Neurology*, **32**, 547–9.

Kulkarni, J., de Castella, A., Smith, D. et al. (1996). A clinical trial of the effects of estrogen in acutely psychotic women. *Schizophr. Res.*, **20**, 247–52.

McCullough, L., Coverdale, J., Bayer, T. et al. (1992). Ethically justified guidelines for family planning interventions to prevent preganancy in female patients with chronic mental illness. *Am. J. Obstet. Gyn.*, **167**, 19–25.

Miller, L. (1997). Sexuality, reproduction, and family planning in women with schizophrenia. *Schizophr. Bull.*, **23**, 623–35.

Miller, L. & Finnerty, M. (1996). Sexuality, pregnancy and childrearing among women with schizophrenia-spectrum disorders. *Psychiatr. Serv.*, **47**, 502–5.

Mogul, K. (1985). Psychological considerations in the use of psychotropic drugs with women patients. *Hosp. Commun. Psychiatry*, **36**, 1080–5.

Morgenstern, H. & Glazer, W. (1993). Identifying risk factors for tardive dyskinesia among long term outpatients maintained with neuroleptic medication. *Arch. Gen. Psychiatry*, **50**, 723–33.

Palmer, S., Lambert, M. & Richards, R. (1991). The MMPI and premenstrual syndrome, profile fluctuations between best and worst times during the menstrual cycle. *J. Clin. Psychol.*, **47**, 215–21.

Preskorn, S. (1993). Recent pharmacological advances in antidepressant therapy for the elderly. *Am. J. Med.*, **94** (suppl. 5A), 2–12.

Raboch, J. (1984). The sexual development and life of female schizophrenic patients. *Arch. Sex. Behav.*, **13**, 341–9.

Ray, W., Griffin, M. & Downey, W. (1989). Benzodiazepines of long and short elimination half-life and the risk of hip fracture. *J.A.M.A.*, **262**, 3303–7.

Riecher-Rössler, A., Häfner, H., Stumbaum, M. et al. (1994). Can oestradiol modulate schizophrenic symptomatology? *Schizophr. Bull.*, **2**, 203–14.

Seeman, M.V. (1983). Interaction of sex, age and neuroleptic dose. *Compr. Psychiatry*, **24**, 125–8.

Seeman, M.V. (1994). Schizophrenic men and women require different treatment programs. *J. Psychiatr. Treat. Eval.*, **5**, 143–8.

Sherwin, S. (1992). *No Longer Patient: Feminist Ethics and Health Care.* Philadelphia: Temple University Press.

Villeneuve, A., Cazejust, T. & Cote, M. (1980). Estrogens in tardive dyskinesia in male psychiatric patients. *Neuropsychobiology*, **6**, 145–51.

Wong, D., Wagner, H.J., Dannals, R. et al. (1984). Effects of age on dopamine and serotonin receptors measured by positron tomography in the living human brain. *Science*, **21**, 1393–6.

Yassa, R. & Jeste, D. (1992). Gender differences in tardive dyskinesia: a critical review of the literature. *Schizophr. Bull.*, **18**, 701–15.

Yonkers, K., Kando, J., Cole, J. et al. (1992). Gender differences in pharmacokinetics and pharmacodynamics of psychotropic medication. *Am. J. Psychiatry*, **149**, 587–95.

9

Overview of sex differences in schizophrenia: where have we been and where do we go from here?

Jill M. Goldstein and Richard R.J. Lewine

This book has presented the reader with an overview of a number of aspects of schizophrenia in women, encompassing biological, psychological and social domains. This chapter provides a synthesis of these findings, making reference to new areas of scientific progress which will further inform our understanding of these issues. The chapter also outlines directions for future research.

Schizophrenia is a heterogeneous disorder. One of the goals of research in this area has been to identify homogeneous subgroups with the assumption that this will lead to the identification of specific aetiological risk factors and focused treatment strategies. Strategies that have been used to identify subtypes of schizophrenia have included grouping patients based on premorbid development, symptom expression, genetic factors, biochemical markers, brain abnormalities, treatment response and course of illness (Goldstein & Tsuang, 1988). Historically, sociodemographic factors, such as one's sex, have not been used to subtype schizophrenia and have been relatively neglected in research on schizophrenia (Wahl & Hunter, 1992). However, over the last 15 years there has been a growing interest in understanding whether, and if so, how one's sex contributes to explaining some of the heterogeneity of the disorder. That is, does one's sex modify the expression of the schizophrenia, and/or contribute to understanding the aetiology of the illness?

The identification of sex differences in schizophrenia is not new, since even Kraepelin described dementia praecox as a disorder primarily afflicting young men (Kraepelin, 1893). The literature, as detailed in this book, shows that men and women with schizophrenia differ regarding age at onset, symptomatology, neurobiological factors, such as brain abnormalities and cognitive function, course of illness, treatment response, incidence and familial transmission. Although there is inconsistency in the literature, many investigators would agree that sex modifies the phenotypic expression of schizophrenia.

However, many would also argue that sex effects seen in schizophrenia are the same as seen in the general population, and therefore one's sex does not contribute to our understanding of the illness. Others have argued that sex is a risk factor, i.e. it has aetiological consequences, for the illness. So, what is the evidence for sex effects in schizophrenia, and is sex a modifier of phenotypic expression or a risk factor for the illness?

Sex and the expression of schizophrenia: age-at-onset, premorbid history, symptomatology

Age-at-onset

As reviewed in Chapter 3, one of the most replicated findings in the schizophrenia literature is the age-at-onset differences between men and women. The literature consistently demonstrates that men have an earlier onset age than women, which is specific to schizophrenia, not an artefact of admission practices, and similar across cultures (Lewine, 1980, 1981; Sartorius et al., 1986; Angermeyer and Kuhn, 1988). The peak period of onset for men is age 18–25 years old and for women, age 25 to mid-30s (Lewine, 1980, 1981; Loranger, 1984; Angermeyer et al., 1989; Goldstein et al., 1989; Hafner et al., 1989). In early adolescence, the onset ratio of men to women is generally 2:1 (Lewine, 1981). However, by age 50 and older, the onset ratio becomes 2:1 female-to-male (Loranger, 1984; Goldstein et al., 1989; Hafner et al., 1989; Castle et al., 1998). Approximately 3–10% of women have onset after age 40, compared to few, if any, men (Lewine, 1981; Angermeyer et al., 1989; Goldstein et al., 1989; Hafner et al., 1989; Castle et al., 1998).

The sex difference in age at onset across studies has been found to depend on the strictness of the diagnostic criteria for defining schizophrenia (Lewine, 1981; Angermeyer and Kuhn, 1988; Hafner et al., 1989). That is, stricter diagnostic criteria result in attenuating the sex difference in age at onset, since one is sampling a more severe group of cases who are more likely to have an earlier age at onset (Lewine et al., 1984; Goldstein, 1995a; see Chapter 3). If women are more likely to have better prognoses and overrepresent less severely ill cases than men (see discussion below), then more severely ill women will be less likely to include later onset women (Goldstein, 1993; Walker & Lewine, 1993).

The magnitude of the age-at-onset sex difference has also been found to vary by geographic region (Angermeyer & Kuhn, 1988). Although women had a later age at onset than men in developing and developed countries in the World Health Organization's study of first-episode schizophrenic cases, the difference was smaller in developing countries (Hambrecht et al., 1992). This may have been due to the fact that few onsets occurred after age 40, which was presumably a consequence of earlier mortality in developing countries (Hambrecht et al., 1992).

Finally, age-at-onset differences by sex are consistently found in studies that specifically controlled for methodological artefacts such as sampling biases. For example, age-at-onset by sex is biased by the underlying age distribution of the population being studied, if men and women in that population have different age distributions (Heimbuch et al., 1980; Chen et al., 1992). Observed sex differences may be a reflection of the differential age distributions rather than sex *per se*. That is, women in general live longer than men, which could result in finding later ages at onset among women than men. Further, sex differences in mortality in schizophrenia may exacerbate the problem (Chen et al., 1992; Goldstein et al., 1992). However, in a study that controlled for the age composition of the population and for differential excess mortality among schizophrenic men and women, sex differences in age at onset remained (Faraone et al., 1994).

As detailed in Chapters 3 and 5, explanations of sex differences in age at onset have ranged from biology to social-role hypotheses (Lewine, 1981, 1988; Seeman, 1982; Castle & Murray, 1991; Castle et al., 1998). It has been hypothesized that sex steroid hormones have a direct effect on age at onset. In rats, estrogens have been found to have a small antidopaminergic effect (Raymond et al., 1978). Thus, it has been hypothesized that estrogens may delay the onset in women. The lowering of estrogens in postmenopausal women could also account for the slight increase in the risk for schizophrenia after age 45 (Lewine, 1981; Seeman, 1982, 1983; Seeman & Lang, 1990; Hafner et al., 1991). In a recent experimental study with neonatal and adult rats, Hafner and colleagues (1991) found that neonatal exposure of estrogen caused a downward regulation of D_2 receptor numbers, which occurred most frequently in the youngest animals. The impact of estrogen on D_2 receptors could contribute to explaining later age at onset in women. An alternative hypothesis is that androgens may trigger earlier onset in men (Lewine, 1981, 1988). Finally, from a social role–social expectations viewpoint of sex differences, it has also been suggested that late adolescence may be a more socially demanding developmental period for boys due to the social expectations of independent work and active courting, thus triggering an earlier onset in men than women (Lewine, 1981; Al-Issa, 1982; Angermeyer & Kuhn, 1988).

Premorbid history

It has been consistently demonstrated across time periods that women tend to have a better premorbid history than men with schizophrenia (Gittelman-Klein & Klein, 1969; Salokangas, 1983; Foerster et al., 1991b; see Chapter 4). Women with schizophrenia are more often married (Watt & Szulecka, 1979; Ciompi, 1980; Wattie & Kedward, 1985; Hafner et al., 1989) and have better childhood histories, including better school achievement and sociability (Gittelman-Klein & Klein, 1969), fewer learning disabilities (Goldstein et al., 1994) and higher IQs (Aylward et al., 1984). Boys at high risk for schizophrenia have exhibited more neurobehavioural deficits than girls at high risk, regarding attentional deficits and neuromotor abnormalities (Mednick et al., 1978; Ehrlenmeyer-Kimling et al., 1984), and aggression (John et al., 1982; Marcus et al., 1987). These studies suggest that males are at higher risk for early developmental deficits than females, prior to the onset of illness, thus indicating a poorer premorbid history. Recent work has shown that the sex difference in premorbid functioning in schizophrenia is specific to schizophrenia, when compared with affective psychoses (Foerster et al., 1991a, 1991b) and not wholly due to sex differences in age at onset (Foerster et al., 1991b).

Symptomatology

The early descriptive literature on schizophrenia suggested that there were sex differences in symptom expression (Cheek, 1964; Lorr & Klett, 1965; Lewine, 1981, 1988). On the inpatient wards, men were described as more passive and withdrawn, and schizoid, while women were described as more explosive, sexually acting out, hostile and agitated, as well as having more affective symptoms in general. Some have argued that results from these earlier studies were in part due to diagnostic misclassification (Lewine et al., 1984), in particular of women who should have been diagnosed as affective psychoses (Lewine, 1981; Lewine et al., 1984; Goldstein & Link, 1988; Goldstein et al., 1990a). A number of studies have shown that the use of more conservative, recent diagnostic criteria differentially excludes more women from the diagnosis than men (Lewine et al., 1984; Goldstein and Link, 1988; Castle et al., 1993). However, in a study of DSM-III-diagnosed patients with schizophrenia, without an age-at-onset limitation, women were still found to express significantly more affective symptoms, paranoia and impulsivity, while men expressed more negative symptoms, such as flat affect (Goldstein & Link, 1988).

The most replicated findings of sex differences in symptomatology have been negative symptoms in men and affective symptoms in women (Lewine, 1981; Walker et al., 1985; Carpenter et al., 1988; Goldstein & Link, 1988; Haas et al., 1988; Copolov et al., 1990; McGlashan & Bardenstein, 1990; Harris et al., 1991; Ring et al., 1991; Hambrecht et al., 1992; Shtasel et al., 1992), even in unmedicated patients (Goldstein & Link, 1988; Shtasel et al., 1992). Regarding positive symptoms, when defined as an overall score, no significant sex differences emerge. However, *specific* positive symptoms have been found to be higher in women, such as more paranoia or persecutory delusions (Goldstein & Link, 1988; Goldstein et al., 1990a; Hambrecht et al., 1992) and auditory hallucinations (Marneros, 1984; Tien, 1991; Rector & Seeman, 1992).

Some have argued that the sex difference in symptom expression in schizophrenia is not specific to schizophrenia (Flor-Henry, 1983). In a study of undergraduates, Raine (1992) showed that women scored significantly higher than men on ideas of reference, odd beliefs, magical thinking and unusual perceptions. Men scored higher on constricted affect and having no close friends (Raine, 1992). This study suggests that sex differences in symptom expression in schizophrenia may be exaggerations of sex differences in normal variants of information processing and social relationships.

Sex, course of illness and treatment response in schizophrenia

Course

As reviewed in Chapter 4, there is a large literature on sex differences in the course and treatment outcomes of schizophrenia. In general, findings show that premenopausal women with schizophrenia experience a better course than men, as defined by rehospitalization, time to relapse, duration of illness, length of hospital stays, response to typical neuroleptics, social adjustment and work functioning (Seeman, 1985; Angermeyer et al., 1989, 1990; McGlashan & Bardenstein, 1990; Seeman & Lang, 1990). However, the longer the observation period, the less marked the treatment outcome difference between the sexes (Goldstein, 1988; Angermeyer et al., 1990; Childers & Harding, 1990; Eaton et al., 1992). This difference may in part be due to the estrogen potentiation of the antipsychotic effect of neuroleptic drugs (Seeman, 1983, 1995; Seeman & Lang, 1990; Riecher-Rossler et al., 1994). Premenopausal women with schizophrenia respond better and to lower doses of typical antipsychotic medications than do men, most likely, in part, due to the antidopaminergic effect of estrogens (Seeman, 1983; Seeman & Lang, 1990). As women age and reach menopause, sex differences in treatment outcomes become attenuated, as estrogen levels drop and women may lose their putative protective effect.

This is in contrast to the studies of sex differences in social adjustment in schizophrenia, which report that women with schizophrenia consistently function better than men, regardless of age (McGlashan & Bardenstein, 1990; Test et al., 1990; Scottish Schizophrenia Research Group, 1992). Findings on sex differences in social adjustment are most likely due to a combination of factors including treatment issues, illness factors, and sex role expectations (Goldstein & Kreisman, 1988; Angermeyer et al., 1989; Haas et al., 1990; Test et al., 1990).

Factors that account for inconsistencies across studies include diagnostic differences, sample selection, differences in lengths of follow-up and in operationalizing dimensions of outcome (Goldstein, 1988, 1995a; Angermeyer et al., 1989). For example, studies that include first-admission patients will demonstrate stronger sex differences in the course of schizophrenia than studies that use multiply hospitalized patients. That is, if women have a better course than men, then a sample of multiply hospitalized cases would differentially exclude women, i.e. the women who recover.

There is a growing body of literature on sex differences in treatment response (Haas et al., 1990; Seeman, 1995; Goldstein et al., 2000), in particular with regard to neuroleptic response. The early work in the area of response to antipsychotic medications, initiated by Seeman (1983), reported that premenopausal women had a more rapid and better treatment response to typical antipsychotic medications than men with schizophrenia, controlling for sex differences in weight (Seeman, 1983; Seeman & Lang, 1990; Hafner et al., 1991; Seeman, 1995; Kulkarni et al., 1996). This was recently challenged (Pinals et al., 1996). Sex differences in treatment, however, dissipated with age, suggesting a protective effect of estrogens, which was withdrawn after menopause. The findings are consistent with animal studies, mentioned earlier in this review, showing the antidopaminergic effects of estrogens (Raymond et al., 1978; DiPaolo et al., 1981; Hafner et al., 1991). Recent clinical studies have suggested significant effects of estrogen levels on symptom exacerbation and treatment response in women with schizophrenia (Hallonquist et al., 1993; Gattaz et al., 1994; Riecher-Rossler et al., 1994; Kulkarni et al., 1996; see Chapter 5). One study has proposed that the higher doses of neuroleptics found among men than women dissipated at later ages due to the changes in testosterone in men rather than estrogens in women (Salokangas, 1995). In addition to the effects of estrogen on treatment response, other pharmacokinetic factors on which men and women differ, such as that women have higher sustained plasma levels, slower gastric absorption, lower protein binding, differential rate of metabolism of drug compounds and differential fat distribution, must be investigated in order to understand sex differences in treatment response (Yonkers et al., 1992).

Atypical antipsychotic medications, i.e. those that do not raise prolactin levels, have been recently developed and marketed. A study of sex differences in response to one atypical antipsychotic medication, clozapine, showed that men with schizophrenia had a better treatment response than women (Lieberman et al., 1994; Szymanski et al., 1996). However, both studies included severely ill, treatment-resistant cases which, as the authors themselves state, could have resulted in a selection bias by sex (Szymanski et al., 1996). That is, as discussed previously, if women are more likely to have a better course and treatment response than men, then treatment-resistant women will be more severely ill than schizophrenic women in general, or than men with schizophrenia. Thus, the finding that women on clozapine had a worse treatment response than men may be a function of selection bias rather than sex *per se.*

In fact, in a recent study comparing olanzapine, another atypical antipsychotic medication, with haloperidol (Goldstein et al., 2000), pre- and postmenopausal women with schizophrenia had at least as good a response to olanzapine as men. Work on sex differences in response to atypical antipsychotic medications is in its infancy. Given that typical and atypical antipsychotic medications are targeted towards different dopamine receptors and other neurotransmitter systems, studies of sex differences in treatment response comparing these types of medications may be fruitful to help us understand the mechanisms by which these medications function as well as the development of sex-specific treatments.

If, as previous literature has shown, there are sex differences in the expression and course of schizophrenia, are there aetiological consequences of this? Areas of research that can contribute to understanding this question are studies of sex differences in incidence, genetic transmission and brain abnormalities.

Sex as a risk factor for schizophrenia

Incidence and prevalence

The incidence of schizophrenia ranges from approximately 0.5 to 2.0 per 10 000 population, and the prevalence from 1 to 12% in different countries. Early work supported the notion that the incidence did not vary by the individual's sex (Neugebauer et al., 1980; Wyatt et al., 1988). However, as discussed in Chapter 3, recent work has challenged this assumption (Sartorius et al., 1986; Cooper et al., 1987; Castle et al., 1991, 1993; Iacono & Beiser, 1992). The difference in findings between the earlier and later studies can in part be explained by the use of different diagnostic criteria. Studies using samples based on DSM-II criteria (American Psychiatric Association, 1968) for schizophrenia included more affective psychosis among women and thus attenuated the sex effect for the incidence of schizophrenia, since women were more likely to express affective disorders than men.

An extensive critical review of the literature on incidence and prevalence of schizophrenia from 1980 to 1994 (Goldstein, 1995a) supported the notion that the sex effect on incidence was, in part, highly dependent on the stringency of the diagnostic criteria and the decision of what other related diagnoses were included in the definition of a case (an idea that was empirically tested by Lewine et al., 1984, Iacono & Beiser, 1992 and Castle et al., 1993). Studies using broader criteria reported no significant sex differences in incidence or prevalence, as did studies that combined schizophrenia with paranoid disorders (Hafner et al., 1989) or other non-affective psychoses (Ring et al., 1991), i.e. disorders in which women have been shown to have higher rates (Orbell et al., 1990; Ring et al., 1991). Studies that used more stringent diagnostic criteria for schizophrenia showed a significant sex effect on incidence, with men experiencing significantly higher rates than women (Lewine et al., 1984; Iacono & Beiser, 1992; Castle et al., 1993). Males younger than age 45 years had the highest incidence compared to young females. Women older than age 45 years had a significantly higher incidence of schizophrenia than men older than age 45 (Goldstein et al., 1989; Iacono & Beiser 1992; Hambrecht et al., 1992; Castle et al., 1991, 1993). However, it was demonstrated in a well-designed population-based study that the higher incidence among older women did not offset the higher incidence among younger males, thus still resulting in a significantly higher rate among men when all ages were combined, e.g. male-to-female risk ratio was 1.34 (Castle et al., 1991, 1993).

Regarding sex differences in prevalence, studies reported a lower male-to-female rate ratio than did incidence studies (Halldin, 1984; Munk-Jørgensen et al., 1986; Freeman & Alport, 1987). However, as with incidence studies, male-to-female rate ratios varied from 1.04 (Bamrah et al., 1981) to 2.1 (Sikanarty & Eaton, 1984), based on diagnostic criteria, sampling frame and duration of the reported prevalence (i.e. point and period, ranging from 2 weeks to lifetime; Goldstein, 1995a). Higher rates among females were also reported in three studies (Nandi et al., 1980; Robins et al., 1984; Bland et al., 1988). However, in these studies, either diagnostic criteria were loosely defined (Nandi et al., 1980) or there was poor diagnostic reliability (Robins et al., 1984). In a well-designed 1-year prevalence study of DSM-III-R schizophrenia cases in a rural area of Ireland, Youseff and colleagues (1991) reported a non-significant male-to-female rate ratio of 1.23, which was replicated in a second study (Youseff et al., 1999). Another recent prevalence study in Ireland, not limited to rural areas, reported a significantly higher prevalence of DSM-III-R (American Psychiatric Association, 1987) schizophrenia among men than women (Kendler et al., 1985).

Prevalence studies are vulnerable to the same methodological artefacts as incidence studies. However, since the estimate of prevalence consists of new cases *and duration*, factors that influence duration in men and women may differ. If the sex difference in incidence reported in current studies is valid, i.e. men have higher rates, then in order for the sex effect on prevalence to dissipate, women would have to have longer durations (i.e. prevalence = incidence × duration). Alternatively, men with schizophrenia may have higher suicide completions than women (Test et al., 1990). It is important in future studies on prevalence or incidence to report the data in such a way as to evaluate the diagnostic issues raised here. Further, as with the incidence findings, the prevalence in young men was found to be higher than in young women, and in older women it was higher than in older men. This attenuated the overall prevalence rates by sex. Future studies need to present age-specific rates by sex in order to answer satisfactorily the question of whether the higher prevalence among older women offsets the higher prevalence among young men. Identifying the significance of sex differences in prevalence is important, since it may have implications for setting parameters in genetic models based on prevalence estimate assumptions.

Genetic transmission

Schizophrenia is a familial disorder, with elevated rates among first-degree relatives ranging from 3% to 15% (Tsuang et al., 1974; Tsuang & Winokur, 1975; Gottesman & Shields, 1982; Kendler et al., 1985). Recent studies have attempted to identify the exact nature of the genetic component. Familial studies have demonstrated that the sex of the proband differentially affects the risk of schizophrenia among first-degree relatives of probands with schizophrenia (Bellodi et al., 1986; Shimizu et al., 1987; Goldstein et al., 1990b; Wolyniec et al., 1992; for a critical review of familial transmission and twin concordance studies (1920–1993), see Goldstein, 1995b). These studies have shown that, compared with relatives of men with schizophrenia, relatives of women have higher rates of schizophrenia and related psychotic spectrum disorders, i.e. schizoaffective and schizophreniform disorders. Relatives of men with schizophrenia have signficantly higher rates of schizotypal personality disorder and flat affect, respectively, a milder expression and subsyndromal phenomenology of the disorder (Goldstein et al., 1990b, Goldstein, 1995b).

The few studies that have attempted to explain the effect of sex on familial risk have looked at age at onset, premorbid history and symptom expression – variables that have been found to differ by sex, as discussed above (Pulver et al., 1990; Goldstein et al., 1992, 1995). Most recent studies have suggested that sex effects may be explained by a pseudoautosomal locus for schizophrenia (Crow, 1988), a dominant X–Y model of transmission (Crow et al., 1994; DeLisi et al., 1994a), genetic heterogeneity (Goldstein et al., 1995) and/or an excess of CAG-based, trinucleotide repeat expansions among female cases (Morris et al., 1995).

For example, the X–Y model of transmission could provide an explanation for sex differences in phenomenology and familial transmission of schizophrenia. A dominant X–Y model of transmission proposes that there are homologous genes on the X and Y chromosomes that contribute to the susceptibility to schizophrenia. Since homologous genes are not identical, their effects on pathophysiology and phenotypic expression are not necessarily identical. Given that women cannot transmit the Y form of the homologous gene, the model also allows for differences in affected relatives based on the sex of the proband.

Another recent family study suggested the possibility that genetic heterogeneity may contribute to explaining sex effects on transmission (Goldstein et al., 1995). Although relatives of females expressed higher rates of the psychotic forms of the schizophrenia spectrum (i.e. schizophrenia, schizoaffective and schizophreniform disorders), relatives of men expressed higher rates of flat affect, i.e. subsyndromal phenomenology that may represent a genetic subform of schizophrenia that is less penetrant for psychosis than other forms (Goldstein et al., 1995). There may be some consistency between expression of schizophrenia and its transmission, since men with schizophrenia exhibit higher rates of flat affect and women exhibit higher rates of persecutory delusions and particular forms of hallucinations (see section on symptomatology, above). This hypothesis has yet to be tested.

Finally, a recent molecular genetic study that tested for trinucleotide repeat expansions in families of schizophrenic patients compared to normal subjects found an excess of CAG repeat size expansions in families of female cases compared to families of normal female subjects and not in male cases compared to their same-sex controls (Morris et al., 1995). These findings suggested a possible genetic abnormality for which women may be at higher risk. Alternatively, the authors stated that the lack of difference among the families of male patients may have been due to the higher rate of CAG expansions among families of male normal controls compared to families of female normal controls. This would be consistent with their finding of no significant sex difference in age at onset in all CAG size categories (Morris et al., 1995).

Sex and brain abnormalities in schizophrenia: normal sexual brain dimorphism

Sex differences in schizophrenia may be due to consequences of the normal sexual dimorphism of the brain, which is described in detail in Chapter 2. Briefly, we will mention a few developmental issues in this chapter since they may provide the basis for understanding sex differences in brain abnormalities in schizophrenia. For example, the pace and timing of grey and white matter development are normally sexually dimorphic in particular brain regions (Jernigan et al., 1991; Benes et al., 1994; Caviness et al., 1996). A number of these areas have also been found to be abnormal in schizophrenia. In animal and human studies, sex hormones have been shown to have permanent organizational effects on brain development, i.e. structural effects established during critical periods of development by genomic and non-genomic events, e.g. regarding neuronal packing density and size, synaptogenesis, cortical maturation, D_2 receptor distribution and density. Sex hormones also have what are called activational effects, which can selectively potentiate neural circuit functions established during development (MacLusky et al., 1987; Naftolin et al., 1990; Witelson et al., 1995). Sexual differentiation of the brain begins during the second trimester of gestation, but extends through early postnatal life to the onset of puberty.

In rodents, aromatase (an enzyme that aromatizes testosterone to estrogen) activity not only occurs in the hypothalamus, but also in cortical and other subcortical areas, i.e. dorsolateral and orbital prefrontal, anterior cingulate, hippocampus and amygdala (MacLusky et al., 1987). This may result in differential growth and maturation of these areas in human boys and girls (MacLusky et al., 1987). Understanding the development and mechanisms of normal sexual dimorphisms can provide clues as to when and where sex may exert its effects on the neurodevelopment of schizophrenia.

As reviewed in Chapter 2, animal and human studies have shown that hormones affect not only grey and white matter development, but also the pace of brain development and asymmetries of brain structures (Geschwind & Galaburda, 1987; Diamond, 1989; Collaer & Hines, 1995). Sex differences in the pace of brain development – slower in males, especially in the left hemisphere, and shown to be hormonally regulated – may place males at higher risk for brain insults that are lateralized and more severe than in females. For example, in humans it has been suggested that testosterone may potentiate the development of the right hemisphere in male fetuses and neonates, whereas female brains develop bilaterally (Geschwind & Galaburda, 1987; Diamond, 1989; Collaer & Hines, 1995). There is some evidence demonstrating that the same prenatal insults can have worse consequences in males than in females, which may be a function of the timing of the insult and differential stages of brain development in boys and girls (Goldman et al., 1974; Ratakallio & Wendt, 1985; Strauss, 1992; Goldstein et al., 1999b).

Sex and cognitive deficits in schizophrenia

Indirect evidence for sex differences in brain abnormalities in schizophrenia comes from studies of cognition. Studies of high-risk children of parents with schizophrenia found that, among high-risk boys versus girls, there were more premorbid neuromotor abnormalities (Erlenmeyer-Kimling et al., 1984), abnormalities of aggression and impulse control and social withdrawal (John et al., 1982; Marcus et al., 1987), lower premorbid IQ (Aylward et al., 1984) and deviant electrodermal response, implicating greater attentional deficits (Mednick et al., 1978). Studies of adults have reported a greater incidence of neurological soft signs and physical anomalies (Green et al., 1987; Murray, 1994) in men with schizophrenia than women, again suggesting an earlier expression of brain damage in men than in women. These studies, along with a recent study of ours (Goldstein et al., 1994), suggest that males with schizophrenia may be at higher risk for more severe consequences from neurodevelopmental deficits than females. This is consistent with the sex ratios found in many other neurodevelopmental disorders, i.e. higher incidence in boys than in girls (Young et al., 1982).

Studies of adults with schizophrenia have suggested that males with schizophrenia showed more neuropsychological deficits compared to male controls (Haas et al., 1990, 1991; Kopala & Clark, 1990; Seidman et al., 1997; Goldstein et al., 1998), including more impairments in verbal intelligence, sustained visual and auditory attention, abstraction, verbal memory, motor function and smell identification than females. In addition, men with schizophrenia who exhibited developmental deficits were particularly impaired on tasks involving verbal processing than women with schizophrenia who had these deficits, suggesting worse consequences for schizophrenia in men than women even when both had developmental deficits (Goldstein et al., 1994). This is consistent with animal and other human studies demonstrating worse consequences for brain abnormalities in males than females if the insults were early in development (Goldman et al., 1974; Ratakallio & Wendt, 1985; Strauss, 1992).

However, the literature on sex differences in cognitive deficits in schizophrenia is inconsistent. A number of studies did not find significant sex differences in cognition (Hoff et al., 1992; Andia et al., 1995; Goldberg et al., 1995; Albus et al., 1997), and still others found that females exhibited greater cognitive deficits than males (Perlick et al., 1992; Lewine et al., 1996). Methodological differences across studies may explain the inconsistencies. These issues will be discussed below, after we discuss the literature on sex differences in structural brain abnormalities, since inconsistencies in both literatures may be explained by similar methodological differences across studies.

Sex and structural brain abnormalities in schizophrenia

Studies on sex differences in structural brain abnormalities in schizophrenia have suggested that there is more pathology among men (Andreasen et al., 1990; Bogerts et al., 1990; Lewine & Seeman, 1995; Goldstein, 1996). However, findings have been inconsistent (Nasrallah et al., 1990; Gur et al., 1991). We would argue that the inconsistencies are due to methodological factors influencing studies of sex differences in brain abnormalities in schizophrenia, such as sample selection and methods for acquiring and analysing brain images (Goldstein, 1996; and see discussion below).

Most of the brain areas implicated in studies of sex differences in schizophrenia are those that have been found to be sexually dimorphic in normals (Pearlson & Pulver, 1994). Men with schizophrenia have been found to have significantly increased cerebrospinal fluid in the lateral ventricles (Andreasen et al., 1990; Flaum et al., 1990; Haas et al., 1991; Nopoulos et al., 1997) and anterior temporal horn (Bogerts et al., 1990) and significant volumetric reductions in medial temporal regions, specifically hippocampus–amygdala (Bogerts et al., 1990), middle and inferior temporal regions (Bryant et al., 1999) and frontal lobe (Andreasen et al., 1994). In addition, more (left) lateralized abnormalities among men have been reported (Bogerts et al., 1990; Cowell et al., 1996) and abnormal torque, reflecting abnormal asymmetric development (Guerguerian & Lewine, 1998). This is also consistent with the prediction that, in normal development, males have a greater vulnerability of the left hemisphere given its slower development in males (Geschwind & Galaburda, 1987; Castle & Murray, 1991). Finally, other abnormalities found preferentially in men with schizophrenia, e.g. increased sulcal volume (Gur et al., 1991) and reduction in thalamic size (Andreasen et al., 1990), suggest more pervasive brain damage in males than females. In contrast, a recent study found greater volume reductions in heteromodal association areas among women with schizophrenia than men (Schlaepfer et al., 1994), areas in which normal women were found to have more grey matter (Schlaepfer et al., 1995).

Sex differences in structural brain asymmetries in schizophrenia have been found in language-associated areas, including the planum temporale, sylvian fissure, superior temporal gyrus, and Heschl's gyrus (Nasrallah, 1986; Falkai et al., 1992; Hoff et al., 1992; Bilder et al., 1994; DeLisi et al., 1994b; Zipursky et al., 1994; Rojas et al., 1997) – again, in areas where asymmetries are found in normal subjects (Kimura, 1983; Kertesz et al., 1990; Reite et al., 1997). Sex differences in brain asymmetries in normal controls and patients may relate to a large body of work demonstrating sex differences in abnormalities in the corpus callosum (for reviews, see Lewine and Seeman, 1995; Woodruff, et al., 1995; see Chapter 2). Some studies have found that males show more deviation from normal subjects (Lewine et al., 1990, 1991) and females show more deviation (Machiyama et al., 1987), both (Casanova et al., 1990; Raine et al., 1990) or neither (Hauser et al., 1989).

In general, findings from previous structural imaging studies lend some support to the hypothesis that sex modifies the phenotypic expression of schizophrenia, since a number of the sex differences in the brain in schizophrenia are exaggerations or attenuations of differences in brain areas that are normally sexually dimorphic (Kimura, 1983; Filipek et al., 1994; Lewine and Seeman, 1995; Goldstein, 1996; Nopoulos et al., 1997). However, there are a number of inconsistencies across studies. Three earlier studies found greater structural abnormalities in women with schizophrenia than men (Nasrallah et al., 1990; Gur et al., 1991; DeLisi et al., 1994b), exhibiting larger lateral and third ventricles, overall ventricular volume and larger posterior temporal horn. Further, a recent study of more severely ill women with schizophrenia showed no significant sex differences in overall cortical grey matter deficits and ventricular size (Lauriello et al., 1997). The lack of finding of significant sex differences in brain abnormalities is typical for many studies. We would argue that the inconsistencies across studies will only be resolved when there is careful consideration of methodological factors that significantly affect the size and significance of sex effects.

Importance of the consideration of specific methodological issues for estimating sex effects in structural and cognitive studies

One reason for the attenuation of the sex effects in the study by Lauriello and colleagues (1997) and others may be the selection of severely ill women in the sample (for discussions of methodological issues, see Goldstein, 1993; 1995a,b; Walker & Lewine, 1993). That is, we and others have shown that women with schizophrenia have better prognoses than men with schizophrenia, i.e. fewer hospitalizations and better psychosocial outcomes (Goldstein, 1988; Angermeyer et al., 1990). A sample of chronically disabled patients with schizophrenia will have excluded individuals who have recovered or have less disability, and these cases are more likely to be women. Thus, a sample of chronically disabled women with schizophrenia is not representative of women with schizophrenia in general. Therefore, within a chronic sample one would expect attenuated sex effects. For example, we have shown that among patients with multiple hospitalizations, sex differences in outcomes were attenuated compared to sex differences in outcomes among first-admission samples of schizophrenics (Angermeyer et al., 1989). Most of the brain imaging studies have used small samples of chronic patients which, we would argue, would result in attenuated sex effects.

For studies of sex differences in cognitive deficits in schizophrenia, regarding selection, it is also important to use patients who are in remission rather than acutely ill. Acutely ill patients will more likely provide information about clinical state differences rather than trait differences. For example, Perlick and colleagues (1992) reported that women with schizophrenia exhibited more severe cognitive deficits than men. However, although they nicely separated their sample into inpatients and outpatients by sex, the inpatient sample included women with schizophrenia who had significantly higher symptom severity than the men with schizophrenia. Thus, the greater severity of cognitive deficits in women could have been due to the severity of illness rather than to sex (Goldstein et al., 1998).

Selection bias may also concern the selection of controls. It is important to match cases to controls, *within sex*, regarding measures typically used for matching, such as premorbid environment/ability and ethnicity. This is important because the size of the sex effects are small, and there is more variability *within* the sexes on measures of brain volumes or functions than *between* the sexes. Thus, closely matching within sex will help to control for extraneous variation that would produce larger standard errors and thus increase type II error (Goldstein et al., 1998).

Finally, with regard to structural imaging studies, the significance of sex effects may be influenced by methods of acquiring images and analysing brain volumes of specific regions of interest. For example, a study by Flaum and colleagues (1995) reported no significant sex differences in volumes of the thalamus, caudate, lenticulate, superior temporal gyrus, and temporal lobe in general. However, the acquisition of image data was in 5 mm slices with 2.5 mm gaps between slices. As the authors themselves state, large non-contiguous slices may produce large partial voluming effects for small brain regions of interest, which result in unreliable volume assessments of small brain regions, thus increasing type II errors.

Functional imaging studies

There is a growing body of functional imaging studies that have specifically examined sex differences in the neural processing of cognitive tasks in normal controls or in persons with schizophrenia. Studies have found that women have approximately 15% higher blood flow and glucose metabolism than men (Gur et al., 1983, 1985; Baxter et al., 1986; Yoshii et al., 1988; Gur & Gur, 1990), which may be due to sex differences in brain weight or brain volume (Yoshii et al., 1988). However, some investigators have shown that there is not a diffuse sex effect on blood flow and glucose metabolism across the entire brain but rather, functional differences in specific brain regions, particularly in the limbic system (Gur et al., 1995). That is, in the resting state, relative metabolism in women versus men was decreased in the lateral and medial temporal lobe and increased in the middle and posterior cingulate, while absolute metabolism was decreased in the occipital–temporal region, temporal pole, hippocampus–amygdala, and orbital prefrontal area (Gur et al., 1995).

In previous work, there were sex differences in asymmetries of function among normal subjects and patients with schizophrenia, in particular when subjects were cognitively challenged (Gur et al., 1983, 1985; Gur & Gur, 1990). Shaywitz and colleagues (1995) demonstrated a sex difference in lateralized activation of the inferior frontal gyri during phonological processing. Studies of normal controls and patients with schizophrenia by Reite and colleagues (1989, 1993) demonstrated further evidence for lateralized brain functioning by sex. Using an auditory evoked potential (EP) paradigm (i.e. tone stimuli), they found sex differences in normal subjects and patients with schizophrenia in the source location of the M-100 EP component, implicating differences in interhemispheric asymmetry in the use of the superior temporal cortex. Women showed bilateral source location for the M-100 component, while in men it was located further anteriorly than in females, particularly on the right. It has been suggested that the M-100 component is most likely localized to cortical areas, including the superior temporal planum and temporoparietal cortex (Reite et al., 1989). In normal controls (Geschwind & Galaburda, 1987) and in patients with schizophrenia (Bogerts et al., 1990; Rossi et al., 1992; DeLisi et al., 1994b; Falkai et al., 1995), these areas, involved in language functions, have been shown to be structurally asymmetrical, i.e. larger on the left.

Where do we go from here?

As detailed in this book, there is now ample evidence to support the hypothesis that schizophrenia is expressed differently in men and women, regarding age at onset, premorbid history, symptom expression and course of illness. Sex differences in the expression of schizophrenia may have aetiological implications, since recent studies have demonstrated a small but significantly higher incidence of schizophrenia among men than women, in particular when stringent criteria for the disorder are applied. Further, the genetic transmission has been found to be influenced by sex. Finally, although still controversial, studies report sex differences in structural and functional brain abnormalities in schizophrenia. The role of sex in understanding the genetics of schizophrenia and brain abnormalities are areas which need further investigation.

Evidence from the animal and human literature clearly demonstrates that the development of the brain differs in males and females, due in large part to the genomic and non-genomic regulatory effects of sex steroid hormones (see Chapter 2). Since schizophrenia is considered, at least in part, to be a neurodevelopmental disorder (Erlenmeyer-Kimling et al., 1984; Marcus et al., 1987; Weinberger, 1987; Murray, 1994; Castle and Murray, 1991), it makes sense that the consequences of early insults to, or genetically determined disruption of, brain development will in some way be influenced by the effects of sex hormones. Thus, one question of interest is whether sex differences in schizophrenia are consequences of the normal sexual brain dimorphism, and whether they are specific to the illness. The evidence to date – although only a small number of studies – suggests that sex differences in brain abnormalities in schizophrenia are, at least in part, consequences of normal sexual brain dimorphism. However, this work is still in its infancy. The use of animal models provides an important contribution to understanding the organizational and activational effects of sex steroid hormones on brain structure and function. Animal studies can be used to test specific hypotheses of interest in schizophrenia about the timing of early brain insults and differential effects on the male and female brain.

The effects of sex steroid hormones on brain function and structure in humans may be suggested by findings in some recent brain imaging studies demonstrating significant effects on brain structure and function of level of masculinity and femininity, irrespective of sex (Weekes et al., 1995; Daniel et al., 1998; Lewine et al. 1999, unpublished data). For example, consistent with others (Gur et al., 1982), early work by Daniel and colleagues (1998) found that women had higher cerebral blood flow than men, particularly in the frontal brain regions. However, they also found that a measure of femininity, independent of sex, significantly predicted higher cerebral blood flow in both 'feminine' women and men. Similarly, Weekes et al. (1995) reported that masculinity, independent of sex, was negatively associated with left ear performance on a dichotic listening task, a measure of functional laterality. This was also supported by a recent structural magnetic resonance imaging study of Lewine and colleagues (1999, unpublished data) who found that feminine male and female subjects, i.e. schizophrenia patients and normal controls, exhibited less lateralization of neuropsychological function, as measured by a dichotic listening task, and larger and rounder corpus callosa than masculine subjects, irrespective of sex. These studies suggest that an understanding of sex differences in brain abnormalities in schizophrenia may involve a broader conceptualization of the meaning of sex and gender, which should be directly tested in future studies of the impact of sex on brain abnormalities in schizophrenia.

Further, the question of interest may not be whether men with schizophrenia have *more* abnormalities than women with schizophrenia, but rather that different brain regions are affected differentially by sex. It is important to identify the specific nature of the sex differences in brain abnormalities in adults with schizophrenia in order to provide clues as to what developmental models might explain these sex effects. For brain imaging studies, this will require segmenting the brain into small, anatomically defined and functionally relevant brain regions in order to investigate abnormalities in specific neural circuits rather than investigations at the lobar level. Further, as found in previous functional imaging studies (Gur et al., 1983, 1985), the question of interest may also be how male and female patients with schizophrenia differentially recruit particular brain regions to perform specific cognitive tasks, in addition to which brain regions are structurally abnormal.

The development of new imaging technologies can contribute valuable information to characterizing these sex differences in schizophrenia. However, one cannot simply separate their data by sex and report whether there are differences or not. This has only added to the confusion in the literature on sex differences in schizophrenia, since the size and significance of sex effects are highly dependent on sampling and other methodological issues in the study design. Publications on sex differences in schizophrenia should be required to specify the characteristics of the patients and controls within sex, for example, with regard to age, parental socioeconomic status, age at onset, number of hospitalizations and duration of illness. Controls should be matched for premorbid environment, i.e. parental socioeconomic status, within sex. Finally, when interpreting the significance or non-significance of one's results, one must think about sample size within sex, since effect sizes by sex are most likely not large. Thus, non-significant results in small sample sizes may be due to low statistical power to find significant effects by sex.

Attention to these methodological considerations will help to clarify the nature of sex effects in schizophrenia and their implications for understanding the aetiology and/or the phenotypic expression of schizophrenia. This may contribute to the development of sex-specific treatments. We would argue that an understanding of sex effects in schizophrenia will also contribute to understanding the impact of sex on other neurodevelopmental disorders, since the sex effects may not be specific to schizophrenia. Further, research in this area will force the field to identify better the nature of *normal* sex differences in brain structures and functions and their relationships to behaviour.

REFERENCES

Albus, M., Hubmann, W., Mohr, F. et al. (1997). Are there gender differences in neuropsychological performance in patients with first episode schizophrenia? *Schizophr. Res.*, **28**, 39–50.

Al-Issa, I. (ed.) (1982). *Gender and Schizophrenia, Gender and Psychopathology*. New York: Academic Press.

American Psychiatric Association (1968). *Diagnostic and Statistical Manual of Mental Disorders*, 2nd edn. Washington, DC: American Psychiatric Association.

Amerian Psychiatric Association (1980). *Diagnostic and Statistical Manual of Mental Disorders*, 3rd edn. Washington, DC: American Psychiatric Association.

American Psychiatric Association (1987). *Diagnostic and Statistical Manual of Mental Disorders*. 3rd edn., revised. Washington, DC: Amerian Psychiatric Association.

Andia, A.M., Zisook, S., Heation, R.K. et al. (1995). Gender differences in schizophrenia. *J. Nerv. Ment. Dis.*, **183**, 522–8.

Andreasen, N.C., Ehrhardt J.C., Swayze, V.W. et al. (1990). Magnetic resonance imaging of the brain in schizophrenia: the pathophysiologic significance of structural abnormalities. *Arch. Gen. Psychiatry.*, **47**, 35–44.

Andreasen, N.C., Flashman, L., Flaum, M. et al. (1994). Regional brain abnormalities in schizophrenia measured with magnetic resonance imaging. *J.A.M.A.*, **272**, 1763–9.

Andreason, P.J., Zametkin, A.J., Guo, A.C., Baldwin, P. & Cohen, R.M. (1994). Gender differences in regional cerebral glucose metabolism in normal volunteers. *Psychiat Res.*, **51**, 175–83.

Angermeyer, M.C., Kuhn, L. (1988). Gender differences in age at onset of schizophrenia. An overview. *Eur. Arch. Psychiatr. Neurol. Sci.*, **237**, 351–64.

Angermeyer, M.C., Goldstein, J.M. & Kuhn, L. (1989). Gender differences in schizophrenia: rehospitalization and community survival. *Psychol. Med.*, **19**, 365–82.

Angermeyer, M.C., Kuhn, L. & Goldstein, J.M. (1990). Gender and the course of schizophrenia: differences in treated outcomes. *Schizophr. Bull.*, **16**, 293–307.

Aylward, E., Walker, E. & Bettes, B. (1984). Intelligence in schizophrenia. *Schizophr. Bull.*, **10**, 430–59.

Bamrah, J.S., Freeman, H.L. & Goldberg, D.P. (1981). Epidemiology of schizophrenia in Salford, 1974–84: changes in an urban community over ten years. *Br. J. Psychiatry*, **159**, 802–10.

Baxter, L.R., Mazziotta, J.C., Phelps, M.E., Selin, C.E., Guze, B.H. & Fairbanks, L. (1986). Cerebral glucose metabolic rates in normal human females versus normal males. *Psychiatry Res.*, **21**, 237–45.

Bellodi, L., Bussoleni, C., Scorza-Smeraldi, R. et al. (1986). Family study of schizophrenia: Exploratory analysis for relevant factors. *Schizophr. Bull.*, **12**, 120–8.

Benes, F.M., Tutle, M., Khan, Y. & Farol, P. (1994). Myelination of a key relay zone in the hippocampal formation occurs in the human brain during childhood, adolescence, and adulthood. *Arch. Gen. Psychiatry*, **51**, 477–84.

Bilder, R.M., Wu, H., Bogerts, B. et al. (1994). Absence of regional hemispheric volume asymmetries in first episode schizophrenia. *Am. J. Psychiatry*, **151**, 1437–47.

Bland, R.C., Orn, H. & Newman, S.C. (1988). Lifetime prevalence of psychiatric disorders in Edmonton. *Acta. Psychiatr. Scand.*, **77**, 24–32.

Bogerts, B., Ashtari, M., Degreef, G., Alvir, J.M.J., Bilder, R.M. & Lieberman, J.A. (1990). Reduced temporal limbic structure volumes on magnetic resonance images in first episode schizophrenia. *Psychiatry Res. Neuroimag.*, **35**, 1–13.

Bryant, N.L., Buchanan, R.W., Vladar, K., Breir, A. & Rothman, M. (1999). Gender differences in temporal lobe structures of patients with schizophrenia: a volumetric MRI study. *Am. J. Psychiatry*, **156**, 603–9.

Carpenter, W.T., Heinrichs, D.W. & Wagman, A.M.I. (1988). Deficit and nondeficit form of schizophrenia: the concept. *Am. J. Psychiatry*, **145**, 578–83.

Casanova, M.F., Sanders, R.D., Goldberg, T.E. et al. (1990). Morphometry of the corpus callosum in monozygotic twins discordant for schizophrenia: A magnetic resonance imaging study. *J. Neurol. Neurosurg. Psychiatry*, **53**, 416–21.

Castle, D.J. & Murray, R. (1991). The neurodevelopmental basis of sex differences in schizophrenia. *Psychol. Med.*, **21**, 565–75.

Castle, D.J., Wessely, S., Der, G. & Murray, R.M. (1991). The incidence of operationally defined schizophrenia in Camberwell 1965–1984. *Br. J. Psychiatry*, **159**, 790–4.

Castle, D.J., Wessely, S. & Murray, R.M. (1993). Sex and schizophrenia: effects of diagnostic stringency, and associations with premorbid variables. *Br. J. Psychiatry*, **162**, 653–64.

Castle, D., Sham, P. & Murray, R. (1998). Differences in distribution of ages of onset in males and females with schizophrenia. *Schizophr. Res.*, **33**, 179–83.

Caviness, V.S., Kennedy, D.N., Richelme, C., Rademacher, J., Filipek, P.A. (1996). The human brain age 7–11 years: a volumetric analysis based upon magnetic resonance images. *Cereb. Cortex*, **6**, 726–36.

Cheek, F.A. (1964). Serendipitous finding: sex roles and schizophrenia. *J. Abnorm. Soc. Psychol.*, **69**, 393–400.

Chen, W.J., Faraone, S.V., Orav, E.J. & Tsuang, M.T. (1992). Estimating age at onset distributions: the bias from prevalent cases and its impact on risk estimation. *Genet. Epidemiol.*, **2**, 219–38.

Childers, S.E. & Harding, C.M. (1990). Gender, premorbid social functioning, and long-term outcome in DSM-III schizophrenia. *Schizophr. Bull.*, **16**, 309–18.

Ciompi, L. (1980). The natural history of schizophrenia in the long-term. *Br. J. Psychiatry*, **136**, 413–20.

Collaer, M.L. & Hines, M. (1995). Human behavioural sex differences: a role for gonadal hormones during early development? *Psychol. Bull.*, **118**, 55–107.

Cooper, J.E., Goodhead, D., Craig, T., Harris, M., Howat, J. & Korer, J. (1987). The incidence of schizophrenia in Nottingham. *Brit. J. Psychiatry.*, **151**, 619–26.

Copolov, D.L., McGorry, P.D., Singh, B.S., et al. (1990). The influence of gender on the classification of psychotic disorders – a multidiagnostic approach. *Acta. Psychiatr. Scand.*, **82**, 8–13.

Cowell, P.E., Kostianovsky, D.J., Gur, R.C., Turetsky, B.I. & Gur, R.E. (1996). Sex differences in neuroanatomical and clinical correlations in schizophrenia. *Am. J. Psychiatry*, **153**, 799–805.

Crow, T.J., DeLisi, L.E., Lofthouse, R. et al. (1994). An examination of linkage of schizophrenia and schizoaffective disorder to the pseudoautosomal region (Xp22.3). *Br. J. Psychiatry*, **164**, 159–64.

Crow, T.J. (1988). Sex chromosomes and psychosis: the case for a pseudoautosomal locus. *Br. J. Psychiatry* **153**, 675–83.

Daniel, D.G., Mathew, R.J., Wilson, W.H. (1998). Sex roles and regional cerebral blood flow. *Psychiatry Res.*, **27**, 55–64.

DeLisi, L.E., Devoto, M., Lofthouse, R. et al. (1994a). Search for linkage to schizophrenia on the X and Y chromosomes. *Am. J. Med. Genet.*, **54**, 113–21.

DeLisi, L.E., Hoff, A.L., Neale, C. & Kushner, M. (1994b). Asymmetries in the superior temporal lobe in male and female first-episode schizophrenic patients: measures of the planum temporale and superior temporal gyrus by MRI. *Schizophr. Res.*, **12**, 19–28.

Diamond, M.C. (1989). Sex and the cerebral cortex. *Biol. Psychiatry*, **25**, 823–5.

DiPaolo, T., Payet, P. & Labrie, F. (1981). Effect of chronic estradiol and haloperidol treatment on striatal dopamine receptors. *Eur. J. Pharmacol.*, **73**, 105–6.

Eaton, W.W., Mortensen, P.B., Herrman, H. et al. (1992). Long-term course of hospitalization. *Schizophr. Bull.*, **18**, 217–28.

Erlenmeyer-Kimling, L., Kestenbaum, C., Bird, H. & Hilldoff, U. (1984). Assessment of the New York high-risk project subjects in sample A who are now clinical deviants. In *Children at Risk for Schizophrenia: A Longitudinal Perspective*, ed. Watt, N., Anthony, N., Wynne, E.J. & Rolf, L.C. Cambridge: Cambridge University Press.

Falkai, P., Bogerts, B., Benno, G. et al. (1992). Loss of sylvian fissure asymmetry in schizophrenia: a quantitative post-mortem study. *Schizophr. Res.*, **7**, 23–32.

Falkai, P., Bogerts, B., Schneider et al. (1995). Disturbed planum temporale asymmetry in schizophrenia. A quantitative post-mortem study. *Schizophr. Res.*, **14**, 161–76.

Faraone, S.V., Chen, W.J. Goldstein, J.M., Tsuang, M.T. (1994) Gender differences in the age at onset of schizophrenia. *Br. J. Psychiatry*, **164**, 625–9.

Filipek, P.A., Richelme, C., Kennedy, D.N. & Caviness, V.S. (1994). The young adult human brain: an MRI-based morphometric study. *Cereb. Cortex.*, **4**, 344–60.

Flaum, M., Arndt, S. & Andreasen, N.C. (1990). The role of ventricle enlargement in schizophrenia: a predominantly male effect. *Am. J. Psychiatry*, **147**, 1327–32.

Flaum, M., Swayze, V.W., O'Leary, D.S. et al. (1995). Effects of diagnosis, laterality, and gender on brain morphology in schizophrenia. *Am. J. Psychiatry.*, **152**, 704–14.

Flor-Henry, P. (1983). The influence of gender on psychopathology. Animal experiments. In *Cerebral Basis of Psychopathology*, ed. Flor-Henry, P. Boston: John Wright PSG.

Foerster, A., Lewis, S.W., Owen, M.J. & Murray, R.M. (1991a). Low birth weight and a family history of schizophrenia predict poor premorbid functioning in psychosis. *Schizophr. Res.*, **5**, 13–20.

Foerster, A., Lewis, S.W., Owen, M.J. & Murray, R.M. (1991b). Pre-morbid adjustment and personality in psychosis: effects of sex and diagnosis. *Br. J. Psychiatry*, **158**, 171–6.

Freeman, H.L. & Alport, M. (1987). Prevalence of schizophrenia in an urban population. *Br. J. Psychiatry*, **149**, 603–11.

Gattaz, W.F., Vogel, P., Riecher-Rossler, A. & Soddu, G. (1994). Influence of the menstrual cycle phase on the therapeutic response in schizophrenia. *Biol. Psychiatry*, **36**, 137–9.

Geschwind, N. & Galaburda, A.M. (1987). *Cerebral Lateralization: Biological Mechanisms, Associations, and Pathology*. Cambridge, MA: MIT Press.

Gittelman-Klein, R. & Klein, D.F. (1969). Premorbid asocial adjustment and prognosis in schizophrenia. *J. Psychiatr. Res.*, **7**, 35–53.

Goldberg, T.E., Gold, J.M., Torrey, E.F. & Weinberger, D.R. (1995). Lack of sex differences in the neuropsychological performance of patients with schizophrenia. *Am. J. Psychiatry*, **152**, 883–8.

Goldman, P.S., Crawford, H.T., Stokes, L.P., Galkin, T.W. & Rosvold, H.E. (1974). Sex-dependent behavioral effects of cerebral cortical lesions in the developing rhesus monkey. *Science*, **186**, 540–2.

Goldstein, J.M. (1988). Gender differences in the course of schizophrenia. *Am. J. Psychiatry*, **145**, 684–9.

Goldstein, J.M. (1993). Impact of sampling biases in explaining discrepancies in studies on gender and schizophrenia: a reply. *Schizophr. Bull.*, **19**, 9–14.

Goldstein, J.M. (1995a). The impact of gender on understanding the epidemiology of schizophrenia. In *Gender and Psychopathology*, ed. M.V. Seeman, pp. 159–99. Washington, DC: American Psychiatric Press.

Goldstein, J.M. (1995b). Gender and the familial transmission of schizophrenia. In *Gender and Psychopathology*, ed. M.V. Seeman. Washington, DC: American Psychiatric Press.

Goldstein, J.M. (1996). Sex and brain abnormalities in schizophrenia: fact or fiction? *Harvard Rev. Psychiatry*, **4**, 110–15.

Goldstein, J.M. & Kreisman, D. (1988). Gender, family environment, and schizophrenia. *Psychol. Med.* **18**, 861–72.

Goldstein, J.M. & Link, B.G. (1988). Gender and the expression of schizophrenia. *J. Psychiatr. Res.*, **22**, 141–55.

Goldstein, J.M. & Tsuang, M.T. (1988). The process of subtyping schizophrenia: strategies in the search for homogeneity. In *Handbook of Schizophrenia*, Vol. 3: *Nosology, Epidemiology, and Genetics*, ed. M.T. Tsuang & J. C. Simpson, pp. 63–83, Amsterdam: Elsevier Science.

Goldstein, J.M., Tsuang, M.T. & Faraone, S.V. (1989). Gender and schizophrenia: implications for understanding the nature of the disorder. *Psychiatr. Res.*, **28**, 243–53.

Goldstein, J.M., Santangelo, S.L., Simpson, J.C. & Tsuang, M.T. (1990a). The role of gender in identifying subtypes of schizophrenia: latent class analytic approach. *Schizophr. Bull.*, **16**, 263–75.

Goldstein, J.M., Faraone, S.V., Chen, W.J., Tolomiczencko, G. & Tsuang, M.T. (1990b). Sex differences in the familial transmission of schizophrenia. *Br. J. Psychiatr.* **156**, 819–26.

Goldstein, J.M., Faraone, S.V., Chen, W.J. & Tsuang, M.T. (1992). Gender and the familial transmission of schizophrenia: Disentangling confounding factors. *Schizophr. Res.*, **7**, 135–40.

Goldstein, J.M., Seidman, L.J., Santangelo, S., Knapp, P. & Tsuang, M.T. (1994). Are schizophrenic men at higher risk for developmental deficits than schizophrenic women? Implications for adult neuropsychological functions. *J. Psychiatr. Res.*, **28** 483–9.

Goldstein, J.M., Faraone, S., Chen, W. & Tsuang, M. (1995). Genetic heterogeneity may in part explain sex differences in the familial risk for schizophrenia. *Biol. Psychiatry*, **38**, 808–13.

Goldstein, J.M., Seidman, L.J., Goodman, J.M. et al. (1998). Are there sex differences in neuropsychological functions among patients with schizophrenia? *Am. J. Psychiatry,* **155**, 1358–64.

Goldstein, J.M., Kennedy, D.N. & Caviness, V.S. (1999). Images in neuroscience. Brain development, XI. Sexual dimorphism. *Am. J. Psychiatry,* **156**, 352.

Goldstein, J.M., Cohen, L.S., Lee, H. et al. (2000). Sex differences in clinical response to the atypical antipsychotic, olanzapine, compared with haloperidol. (under review).

Gottesman, I.I. & Shields, J. (1982). *The Epigenetic Puzzle,* Cambridge: Cambridge University Press.

Green, M.F., Satz, P., Soper, H.V. & Kharabi, F. (1987). Relationship beween physical anomalies and age at onset of schizophrenia. *Am. J. Psychiatry,* **144**, 666.

Guerguerian, R. & Lewine, R.R.J. (1998). Brain torque and sex differences in schizophrenia. *Schizophr. Res.,* **30**, 175–81.

Gur, R.E., Gur, R.C. (1990). Gender differences in regional cerebral blood flow. *Schizophr. Bull.,* **16**, 247–54.

Gur, R.C., Gur, R.E., Obrist, W.D. et al. (1982). Sex and handedness differences in cerebral blood flow during rest and cognitive activity. *Science,* **217**, 659–61.

Gur, R.E., Skolnick, B.E., Gur, R.C. et al. (1983). Brain function in pscyhiatric disorders: I. Regional cerebral blood flow in medicated schizophrenics. *Arch. Gen. Psychiatry,* **40**, 1250–4.

Gur, R.E., Gur, R.C., Skolnick, B.E. et al. (1985). Brain function in psychiatric disorders: III. Regional cerebral blood flow in unmedicated schizophrenics. *Arch. Gen. Psychiatry,* **42**, 329–34.

Gur, R.E., Mozley, P.D., Resnick, S.M. et al. (1991). Magnetic resonance imaging in schizophrenia: I. Volumetric analysis of brain and cerebrospinal fluid. *Arch. Gen. Psychiatry,* **48**, 407–12.

Gur, R.C., Mozley, L.H., Mozley, P.D., et al. (1995). Sex differences in regional cerebral metabolism during a resting state. *Science,* **267**, 528–31.

Haas, G.L., Glick, I.D., Clarkin, J.F. et al. (1988). Inpatient family intervention: A randomized clinical trial. II: Results at hospital discharge. *Arch. Gen. Psychiatry,* **45**, 217–24.

Haas, G.L., Glick, I.D., Clarkin, J.F., Spencer, J.H. & Lewis, A.B. (1990). Gender and schizophrenia outcome: a clinical trial of an inpatient family intervention. *Schizophr. Bull.,* **16**, 277–92.

Haas, G.L., Sweeney, J.A., Hien, D.A., Goldman, D. & Deck, M. (1991). Gender differences in schizophrenia [abstract and presentation]. *Schizophr. Res.,* **4**, 277.

Hafner, H., Riecher, A., Maurer, K. et al. (1989). How does gender influence age at first hospitalization for schizophrenia? A transnational case register study. *Psychol. Med.,* **19**, 903–18.

Hafner, H., Behrens, S., De Vry, J. & Gattaz, W.F. (1991). An animal model for the effects of estradiol on dopamine-mediated behavior: implication for sex differences in schizophrenia. *Psychiatry Res.*, **38**, 125–34.

Halldin, J. (1984). Prevalence of mental disorder in an urban population in central Sweden. *Acta. Psychiatr. Scand.*, **69**, 503–18.

Hallonquist, J., Seeman, M.V., Lang, M. & Rector, N.A. (1993). Variation in symptom severity over the menstrual cycle of schizophrenics. *Biol. Psychiatry*, **33**, 207–9.

Hambrecht, M., Maurer, K., Sartorius, N. & Hafner, H. (1992). Transnational stability of gender differences in schizophrenia? An analysis based on the WHO study on determinants of outcome of severe mental disorders. *Eur. Arch. Psychiatry Clin. Neurosci.*, **242**, 6–12.

Harris, M.J., Jeste, D.V., Krull, A. et al. (1991). Deficit syndrome in older schizophrenic patients. *Psychiatry Res.*, **39**, 285–92.

Hauser, P., Dauphinais, I.D., Berrettini, W., DeLisi, L.E., Gelernter, J. & Post, R.M. (1989). Corpus callosum dimensions measured by magnetic resonance imaging in bipolar affective disorder and schizophrenia. *Biol. Psychiatry*, **26**, 659–68.

Heimbuch, R.C., Matthysse, S. & Kidd, K.K. (1980). Estimating age of onset distributions for disorders with variable onset. *Am. J. Hum. Genet.*, **32**, 564–74.

Hoff, A.L., Riordan, H., O'Donnell, D. et al. (1992). Anomalous lateral sulcus asymmetry and cognitive funciton in first-episode schizophrenia. *Schizophr. Bull.*, **18**, 257–72.

Iacono, W.G. & Beiser, M. (1992). Are males more likely than females to develop schizophrenia? *Am. J. Psychiatry.* **149**, 1070–4.

Jernigan, T.L., Trauner, D.A., Hesselink, J.R. & Tallal, P.A. (1991). Maturation of human cerebrum observed *in vivo* during adolescence. *Brain*, **114**, 2037–949.

John, R., Mednick, S.A. & Schulsinger, F. (1982). Teacher reports as predictors of schizophrenia and borderline schizophrenia: a Bayesian decision analysis. *J. Abnorm. Psychol.*, **143**, 383–8.

Kendler, K.S., Gruenberg, A.M. & Tsuang, M.T. (1985). Psychiatric illness in first-degree relatives of schizophrenia and surgical control patients. *Arch. Gen. Psychiatry*, **42**, 770–9.

Kertesz, A., Polk, M. & Black, S.E.J.H. (1990). Sex, handedness, and the morphometry of cerebral asymmetries on magnetic resonance imaging. *Brain Res.*, **530**, 40–8.

Kimura, D. (1983). Sex differences in cerebral organization for speech and praxic functions. *Can. J. Psychol.*, **37**, 19–35.

Kopala, L. & Clark, C. (1990). Implications of olfactory agnosia for understanding sex differences in schizophrenia. *Schizophr. Bull.*, **16**, 255–61.

Kraepelin, E. (1893). *Dementia Praecox and Paraphrenia*. Translated by R.M. Barclay. Facsimile 1919 edition. New York: R. Kreiger.

Kulkarni, J., De Castella, A., Smith, D., Taffe, J., Keks, N. & Copolov, D. (1996). A clinical trial of the effects of estrogen in acutely psychotic women. *Schizophr. Res.*, **20**, 247–52.

Lauriello, J., Hoff, A., Wieneke, M.H. et al. (1997). Similar extent of brain dysmorphology in severely ill women and men with schizophrenia. *Am. J. Psychiatry*, **154**, 819–25.

Lewine, R.R.J. (1980). Sex differences in age of symptom onset and first hospitalization in schizophrenia. *Am. J. Orthopsychiatry*, **50**, 316–22.

Lewine, R.R.J. (1981). Sex differences in schizophrenia. Timing or subtypes? *Psych. Bull.*, **90**, 432–44.

Lewine, R.R.J. (1988). Gender and schizophrenia. In *Handbook of Schizophrenia*, ed. M.T. Tsuang & J.C. Simpson, vol. 3. pp. 379–97. Amsterdam: Elsevier.

Lewine, R.R.J. & Seeman, M.V. (1995). Gender, brain and schizophrenia: anatomy of differences/differences of anatomy. In *Gender and Psychopathology*, ed. M.V. Seeman, pp. 131–58. Washington, DC: American Psychiatric Press.

Lewine, R.R.J., Burback, D. & Meltzer, H.Y. (1984). Effect of diagnostic criteria on the ratio of male to female schizophrenic patients. *Am. J. Psychiatry*, **141**, 84–7.

Lewine, R.R.J., Gulley, L.R., Risch, S.C., Jewart, R. & Houpt, J.L. (1990). Sexual dimorphism, brain morphology, and schizophrenia. *Schizophr. Bull.*, **16**, 195–203.

Lewine, R.J., Flashman, L., Gulley, L. et al. (1991). Sexual dimorphism in corpus callosum and schizophrenia. *Schizophr. Res.*, **4**, 63–4.

Lewine, R.R.J., Walker, E.F., Shurett, R., Caudle, J. & Haden, C. (1996). Sex differences in neuropsychological functioning among schizophrenic patients. *Am. J. Psychiatry*, **153**, 1178–84.

Lieberman, J. A., Safferman, A.Z., Pollack, S. et al. (1994). Clinical effects of clozapine in chronic schizophrenia: response to treatment and predictors of outcome. *Am. J. Psychiatry*, **151**, 1744–52.

Loranger, A.W. (1984). Sex difference in age at onset of schizophrenia. *Arch. Gen. Psychiatry*, **41**, 157–61.

Lorr, M. & Klett, C.J. (1965). Constancy of psychotic syndromes in men and women. *J. Consult. Clin. Psychol.*, **29**, 309–13.

MacLusky, N.J., Clark, A.S., Naftolin, F. & Goldman-Rakic, P.S. (1987). Estrogen formation in the mammalian brain: possible role of aromatase in sexual differentiation of the hippocampus and neocortex. *Steroids*, **50**, 4–6.

Machiyama, Y., Watanabe, Y. & Machiyama, R. (1987). Neuroanatomical studies of the corpus callosum in schizophrenia: evidence of aberrant interhemispheric fiber connection. In *Cerebral Dynamics, Laterality, and Psychopathology*, eds. R. Takahashi, P. Flor-Henry, J. Gruzelier & S. Niwa, pp. 411–12. New York: Elsevier Press.

Marcus, J., Hans, S.L., Nagler, S., Auerbach, J.G., Mirsky, J. & Aubrey, A. (1987). Review of the NIMH Israeli Kibbutz-City study and the Jerusalem infant development study. *Schizophr. Bull.*, **13**, 425–38.

Marneros, A. (1984). Frequency of occurrence of Schneider's first rank symptoms in schizophrenia. *Eur. Arch. Psychiatry Neurol. Sci.*, **234**, 78–82.

McGlashan, T.H. & Bardenstein, K.K. (1990) Gender differences in affective, schizoaffective, and schizophrenic disorders. *Schizophr. Bull.* **16**, 319–29.

Mednick, S.A., Schulsinger, F., Teasdale, T.W., Schulsinger, H., Venables, P.H. & Rock, D.R. (1978). Schizophrenia in high-risk children: sex differences in predisposing factors. In *Cognitive Defects in the Development of Mental Illness*, ed. G. Serban, pp. 169–97. New York: Brunner/Mazel.

Morris, A.G., Gaitonde, E., McKenna, P.J., Mellon, J.D. & Hunt, D.M. (1995). CAG repeat expansions and schizophrenia: associated with disease in females and with early age at onset. *Hum. Mol. Genet.* **4**, 1957–61.

Munk-Jørgensen, P., Weeke, A., Jensen, E.B., Dupont, A. & Stromgren, E. (1986). Changes in utilization of Danish psychiatric institutions, II: Census studies 1977 and 1982. *Compr. Psychiatry*, **27**, 416–29.

Murray, R.M. (1994) Neurodevelopmental schizophrenia: the rediscovery of dementia praecox. *Br. J. Psychiatry* **165**, 6–12.

Murray, R.M., O'Callaghan, E., Castle, D.J. & Lewis, S.W. (1992). A neurodevelopmental approach to the classification of schizophrenia. *Schizophr. Bull.* **18**, 319–32.

Naftolin, F., Garcia-Segura, L.M. & Keefe, D. (1990). Estrogen effects on the synaptology and neural membranes of the rat hypothalamic arcuate nucleus. *Biol. Reprod.* **42**, 21–8.

Nandi, D.N., Mukherjee, S.P., Boral, G.C. et al. (1980). Socio-economic status and mental morbidity in certain tribes and castes in India: a cross-cultural study. *Br. J. Psychiatry*, **136**, 73–85.

Nasrallah, H.A (1986). Cerebral hemisphere asymmetries and interhemispheric integration in schizophrenia. In *Handbook of Schizophrenia*, vol. 1. *The Neurology of Schizophrenia*, ed. H.A. Nasrallah & D.R. Weinberger, pp. 157–74. Amsterdam: Elsevier.

Nasrallah, H.A., Schwartzkopf, S.B., Olson, S.C. & Coffman, J.A. (1990). Gender differences in schizophrenia on MRI brain scans. *Schizophr. Bull.* **16**, 205–10.

Neugebauer, R., Dohrenwend, P.R. & Dohrenwend, B.S. (1980). Formulation of hypotheses about the true prevalence of functional psychiatric disorders among adults in the U.S. In: Dohrenwend, B.P., Dohrenwend, B.S., Gould, M. et al. (eds) *Mental Illness in the United States: Epidemiological Estimates*. New York: Prager, pp. 45–94.

Nopoulos, P., Flaum, M. & Andreasen, N.C. (1997). Sex differences in brain morphology in schizophrenia. *Am. J. Psychiatry*, **154**, 1648–54.

Orbell, S., Trew, K. & McWhirter, L. (1990). Mental illness in Northern Ireland. A comparison with Scotland and England. *Soc. Psychiatry Psychiatr. Epidemiol.*, **25**, 165–9.

Pearlson, G.D. & Pulver, A.E. (1994). Sex, schizophrenia and the cerebral cortex. In *Schizophrenia: Exploring the Spectrum of Psychosis*, ed. R.J. Ancill, S. Holliday & J. Higenbottam, pp. 345–62. Chichester: John Wiley.

Perlick, D., Mattis, S., Stastny, P. & Teresi, J. (1992). Gender difference cognition in schizophrenia. *Schizophr. Res.* **8**, 69–73.

Pinals, D.A., Malhotra, A.K., Missar, C.D., Pickar, D. & Breier, A. (1996). Lack of gender differences in neuroleptic response in patients with schizophrenia. *Schizophr. Res.* **22**, 215–22.

Pulver, A.E., Brown, C.H., Wolyniec, P. et al. (1990). Schizophrenia: age at onset, gender, and familial risk. *Acta Psychiatr. Scand.*, **82**, 344–51.

Raine, A. (1992). Sex differences in schizotypal personality in a nonclinical population. *J Abnorm. Psychol.*, **101**, 361–4.

Raine, A., Harrison, G.N., Reynolds, G.P., Sheard, C., Cooper, J.E. & Medley, I. (1990). Structural and functional characteristics of the corpus callosum in schizophrenics, psychiatric controls, and normal controls. *Arch. Gen. Psychiatry*, **47**, 1060–4.

Ratakallio, P. & Wendt, L.V. (1985). Prognosis for low birth weight infants up to the age of 14. *Dev. Med. Child. Neurol.* **27**, 655.

Raymond, V., Beaulieu, M., Labrie, F. & Boissier, J. (1978). Potent antidopaminergic activity of estradiol at the pituitary level on prolactin release. *Science*, **200**, 1173–5.

Rector, N.A. & Seeman, M.V. (1992). Auditory hallucinations in women and men. *Schizophr. Res.*, **7**, 233–6.

Reite, M., Teale, P., Goldstein, L., Whalen, J. & Linnville, S. (1989). Late auditory magnetic sources may differ in the left hemisphere of schizophrenic patients. *Arch. Gen. Psychiatry*, **46**, 565–72.

Reite, M., Cullum, C.M., Stocker, J., Teale, P. & Kozora, E. (1993). Neuropsychological test performance and MEG-based brain lateralization: sex differences. *Br. Res. Bull.*, **32**, 325–8.

Reite, M. Sheeder, J., Teale, P. et al. (1997). Magnetic source imaging evidence of sex differences in cerebral lateralization in schizophrenia. *Arch. Gen. Psychiatry*, **54**, 433–40.

Riecher-Rossler, A., Hafner, H., Stumbaum, M., Maurer, K. & Shmidt, R. (1994). Can estradiol modulate schizophrenic symptomatology? *Schizophr. Bull.*, **20**, 203–13.

Ring, N., Tantam, D., Montague, L. et al. (1991). Gender differences in the incidence of definite schizophrenia and atypical psychosis – focus on negative symptoms of schizophrenia. *Acta. Psychiatr. Scand.*, **84**, 489–96.

Robins, L.N., Helzer, J.E., Weissman, M.M. et al. (1984). Lifetime prevalence of specific psychiatric disorders in three sites. *Arch. Gen. Psychiatry*, **41**, 949–58.

Rojas, D.C., Teale, P., Sheeder, J., Simon, J. & Reite, M. (1997). Sex-specific expression of Heschl's gyrus functional and structural abnormalities in paranoid schizophrenia. *Am. J. Psychiatry*, **154**, 1655–62.

Rossi, A., Stratta, P., Mattei, P. et al. (1992). Planum temporale in schizophrenia: A magnetic resonance study. *Schiz. Res.*, **7**, 19–22.

Salokangas, R.K.R. (1983). Prognostic implications of the sex of schizophrenic patients. *Br. J. Psychiatry*, **142**, 145–51.

Salokangas, K.R. (1995). Gender and the use of neuroleptics in schizophrenia – further testing of the estrogen hypothesis. *Schiz. Res.*, **16**, 7–16.

Sartorius, N., Jablensky, A., Korten, A. et al. (1986). Early manifestations and first-contact incidence of schizophrenia in different cultures. *Psych. Med.*, **16**, 909–28.

Schlaepfer, T.E., Harris, G.J., Tien, A.Y. et al. (1994). Decreased regional cortical gray matter volume in schizophrenia. *Am. J. Psychiatry*, **151**, 842–8.

Schlaepfer, T.E., Harris, G.J., Tien, A.Y., Peng, L., Lee, S. & Pearlson, G.D. (1995). Structural differences in the cerebral cortex of healthy female and male subjects: a magnetic resonance imaging study. *Psychiatr. Res. Neuroimaging*, **61**, 129–35.

Scottish Schizophrenia Research Group (1992). The Scottish first episode schizophrenia study. VIII. Five-year follow-up: clinical and psychosocial findings. The Scottish Schizophrenia Research Group. *Br. J. Psychiatry*, **161**, 496–500.

Seeman, M.V. (1982). Gender differences in schizophrenia. *Can. J. Psychiatry*, **27**, 107–11.

Seeman, M.V. (1983). Interaction of sex, age, and neuroleptic dose. *Comp. Psychiatry*, **24**, 125–8.

Seeman, M.V. (1985). Sex and schizophrenia. *Can. J. Psychiatry*, **30**, 313–15.

Seeman, M.V. (1995). Gender differences in treatment response in schizophrenia. In *Gender and Psychopathology*, ed. M.V. Seeman, pp. 227–51. Washington DC: American Psychiatric Press.

Seeman, M.V. & Lang, M. (1990). The role of estrogens in schizophrenia gender differences. *Schizophr. Bull.*, **16**, 185–94.

Seidman, L.J., Goldstein, J.M., Goodman, J.M. et al. (1997). Sex differences in olfactory identification and Wisconsin Card Sorting performance in schizophrenia: relationship to attention and verbal ability. *Biol. Psychiatry*, **42**, 104–15.

Shaywitz, B.A., Shaywitz, S.E., Pugh, K.R. et al. (1995). Sex differences in the functional organization of the brain for language. *Nature*, **373**, 607–9.

Shimizu, A., Massayoshi, K., Yamaguchi, N., et al. (1987). Morbidity risk of schizophrenia to parents and siblings of schizophrenic patients. *Jpn. J. Psychiatry Neurol.*, **41**, 65–70.

Shtasel, D.L., Gur, R.E., Gallacher, F., Heimberg, C., Gur, R.C. (1992). Gender differences in the clinical expression of schizophrenia. *Schizophr. Res.*, **7**, 225–31.

Sikanarty, T. & Eaton, W.W. (1984). Prevalence of schizophrenia in the Labadi district of Ghana. *Acta. Psychiatr. Scand.*, **69**, 156–61.

Strauss, E. (1992). Sex-related differences in the cognitive consequences of early left-hemispheric lesions. *J. Clin. Exp. Neuropsychol.*, **14**, 738–48.

Szymanski, S., Lieberman, J., Pollack, S. et al. (1996). Gender differences in neuroleptic nonresponsive clozapine-treated schizophrenics. *Biol. Psychiatry*, **39**, 249–54.

Test, M.A., Burke, S.S. & Wallisch, L.S. (1990). Gender differences of young adults with schizophrenic disorders in community care. *Schizophr. Bull.*, **16**, 331–44.

Tien, A.Y. (1991). Distribution of hallucinations in the population. *Soc. Psychiatry Psychiatr. Epidemiol.*, **26**, 287–92.

Tsuang, M.T. & Winokur, G. (1975). The Iowa-500: field work in a 35–year follow-up of depression, mania, and schizophrenia. *Can. Psychol. Assoc. J.*, **20**, 359–65.

Tsuang, M.T., Fowler, R.C., Cadoret, R.J. & Monnelly, E. (1974). Schizophrenia among first-degree relatives of paranoid and nonparanoid schizophrenics. *Compr. Psychiatry*, **15**, 295–302.

Wahl, O.F. & Hunter, J. (1992). Are gender effects being neglected in schizophrenia research? *Schizophr. Bull.*, **18**, 313–18.

Walker, E.F., Lewine, R.R.J. (1993). Sampling biases in studies of gender and schizophrenia. *Schizophr. Bull.*, **19**, 1–7.

Walker, E., Bettes, B.A., Kain, E.L. et al. (1985). Relationship of gender and marital status with symptomatology in psychotic patients. *J. Abnorm. Psychol.*, **94**, 42–50.

Watt, D.C. & Szulecka, T.K. (1979). The effect of sex, marriage and age at first admission on the hospitalization of schizophrenics during two years following discharge. *Psychol. Med.*, **9**, 529–39.

Wattie, B.J.S. & Kedward, H.B. (1985). Gender differnces in living conditions found among male and female schizophrenic patients on a follow-up study. *Int. J. Soc. Psychiatry*, **31**, 205–16.

Weekes, N.Y., Zaidel, D.W. & Zaidel, E. (1995). The effects of sex and sex role attribution on the ear advantage in dichotic listening. *Neuropsychology*, **9**, 62–7.

Weinberger, D.R. (1987). Implications of normal brain development for the pathogenesis of schizophrenia. *Arch. Gen. Psychiatry*, **44**, 660–9.

Witelson, S.F., Glezer, I.I. & Kigar, D.L. (1995). Women have greater density of neurons in posterior temporal cortex. *J. Neurosci.*, **15**, 3418–28.

Wolyniec, P.S., Pulver, A.E., McGrath, J.A., et al. (1992). Schizophrenia: gender and familial risk. *J. Psychiatr. Res.*, **26**, 17–27.

Woodruff, P.W.R., McManus, I.C. & David, A.S. (1995). A meta-analysis of corpus callosum size in schizophrenia. *J. Neurol. Neurosurg. Psychiatry*, **58**, 457–61.

Wyatt, R.J. Alexander, R.C. Egan, M.F. & Kirch, D.G. (1988). Schizophrenia, just the facts: what we know, how well do we know it? *Schizophr. Res.*, **1**, 3–18.

Yonkers, K.A., Kando, J.C., Cole, J.O. & Blumenthal, S. (1992). Gender differences in pharmokinetics and pharmacodynamics of psychotropic medication. *Am. J. Psychiatry*, **149**, 587–95.

Yoshii, F., Barker, W.W., Chang, J.Y. et al. (1988). Sensitivity of cerebral glucose metabolism to age, gender, brain volume, brain atrophy, and cerebrovascular risk factors. *J. Cereb. Blood Flow Metab.*, **8**, 654–61.

Young, J.G., Cohen, D.J., Shaywitz, S.E. et al. (1982). Assessment of brain function in clinical pediatric research: behavioral and biological strategies. *Schizophr. Bull.* **8**, 205–35.

Youseff, H.A., Kinsella, A. & Waddington, J.L. (1991). Evidence for geographical variations in the prevalence of schizophrenia in rural Ireland. *Arch. Gen. Psychiatry*, **48**, 254–8.

Youssef, H.A., Scully, P.J., Kinsella, A. & Waddington, J.L. (1999). Geographical variation in rate of schizophrenia in rural Ireland by place at birth vs place at onset. *Schizophr. Res.*, **37**, 233–43.

Zipursky, R.B., Marsh, L., Lim, K.O. et al. (1994). Volumetric MRI assessment of temporal lobe structures in schizophrenia. *Biol. Psychiatry*, **35**, 501–16.

Index